The Medical
Discoveries of
EDWARD BACH,
Physician

*Other Keats Titles on the Work
of Dr. Edward Bach*

The Medical Discoveries of EDWARD BACH, Physician

Nora Weeks

Keats Publishing, Inc. New Canaan, Connecticut

The Medical Discoveries of Edward Bach, Physician is not intended as medical advice. Its intent is solely informational and educational. Please consult a health professional should the need for one be indicated.

THE MEDICAL DISCOVERIES OF EDWARD BACH, PHYSICIAN

Fourth printing, January 1994

ISBN: 0-87983-642-3

Library of Congress Card Catalog Number 79-88118

Printed in the United States of America

Published by Keats Publishing, Inc.
27 Pine Street (Box 876)
New Canaan, Connecticut 06840-0876

CONTENTS

CHAPTER		PAGE
I	Edward Bach. Early years	9
II	1903-1906. Experience in the Bach brass foundry	12
III	Medical Training	15
IV	Pathologist and bacteriologist	19
V	Homœopathy. The Bach Nosodes . .	25
VI	1922-1928. The Seven Bach Nosodes (continued)	32
VII	1928-1930. The beginning of the new work and the finding of the first three herbal remedies . .	39
VIII	1930. The last weeks in London . .	44
IX	May-July 1930. Wales. The discovery of the 'sun method' of preparing the new remedies . .	48
X	1930. June and July. The writing of the book *Heal Thyself*	53
XI	1930. August. Cromer. The principles of the new method of treatment	57
XII	1930. August and September. The finding and preparing of seven of the new remedies . . .	64
XIII	The winter of 1930. The publishing of the book *Heal Thyself*. Some results obtained with the new remedies, taken from Edward Bach's case book .	70
XIV	1931-1932. The finding and preparing of the last three remedies of the *Twelve Healers* series. The writing of the book *Free Thyself* . . .	80
XV	Winter 1932. Cromer. The correspondence with the General Medical Council. Reports of cases treated with the three remedies: Water Violet, Rock Rose and Gentian	85
XVI	1933. Marlow. Cromer. The publishing of the pamphlet *The Twelve Healers*, and the finding and preparation of the remedies called 'The Four Helpers'	94
XVII	1933-1934. The last year at Cromer. The publishing of *The Twelve Healers and Four Helpers*. The preparing of the remedies Oat, Olive and Vine . . .	101
XVIII	Cromer. 1930-1934.	106

CHAPTER   PAGE

XIX   1934-1935. Sotwell. The book *The Twelve Healers and Seven Helpers*. The finding of the new nineteen remedies 111

XX   Sotwell. The book *The Twelve Healers and Other Remedies*. The lecture 'The Healing Herbs.' Last illness and death of Edward Bach. .   .   . 119

XXI   Results obtained by the thirty-eight herbal remedies 124

XXII   Edward Bach: Personal impressions .   .   . 134

EDWARD BACH

Eager and ardent, like a living flame,
  Without a thought of self, desiring ever
Nor wealth nor power nor influence nor fame
  Except as those might forward his endeavour
To help mankind. So swift to understand
  All doubts and fears and failures, yet so slow
To judge or to condemn, he set his hand
  Alone to heal, to help those powers to grow
That make for fellowship and cast out hate
  And aim to help the whole wide world to gain
Touch with the Infinite. Darkly we wait
  So long for light, so oft it seems in vain,
But here was a life that sped too swiftly by
Yet kindled fires that will be slow to die.

C.E.W.

"The physician's high and only mission is to restore the sick to health, to cure . . ." —Hahnemann.

CHAPTER I

EDWARD BACH. EARLY YEARS

EDWARD BACH was born on September 24th, 1886, at Moseley, a village about three miles outside Birmingham in Warwickshire, and was the eldest of a family of two boys and a girl.

He was a delicate baby, and was only with much care brought through the difficult first years of his life, though as he grew older his health improved.

As a boy his determination and intensity of purpose were outstanding; he possessed such power of concentration that he became absorbed in anything that interested him, allowing nothing to distract his attention or to interfere with his purpose.

He was full of vitality and love of adventure, good at games and ready for any mischief and, thanks to the Welsh strain in his blood, acutely intuitive and sensitive.

All that pertained to Wales had a great attraction for him; his own family, as the name Bach implies, came from that land many years ago, and his intuitive, idealistic nature, his love of all beauty, his beautiful speaking voice marked him a true son of that mystic land.

Howard Fisher, the Head of Winterloe School, Moseley, where he was educated, was a Welshman, and for him Edward Bach had a great affection which lasted in after years. He would often tell of the half-holiday he had earned as a reward for spelling Caernarvon with an 'e,' and the joy it had given to his Welsh master.

This love of Wales drew Edward Bach to her again and again. When he was a schoolboy he would spend his holidays tramping through the Welsh villages and over the mountains, sleeping each night where he could, happy in the company of his friends the birds and trees and wild flowers, for his love of Nature showed itself at a very early age.

Later on he was to find, near one of the mountain rivers, the first of the herbal remedies for which he is famous; and later still, in the peace and quiet of a Welsh village, he was to work out the principles of the new system of herbal medicine.

His was a many-sided nature. Independent and positive from his earliest years, endowed with a great sense of humour and fun, he would at times become silent and meditative, roaming the countryside alone, or sitting and gazing at the wonders of a few yards of grassy bank or the bark of some big tree for hours at a time.

Any human being, bird or creature in pain or distress aroused in him such compassion and desire to help their suffering that he determined, whilst still a boy at school, to be a doctor.

This overwhelming compassion for others, which gave him so great an understanding of their distress, was one of his most striking qualities, and one which made him beloved by all who came in contact with him.

He would oftentimes sit in the school classroom and dream of the time when he might begin his work. He would dream that he had found some simple form of healing which would cure all forms of disease. He would also dream that healing power flowed from his hand and that all whom he touched were healed; and these were no schoolboy flights of imagination, but the inner knowledge of what was to come to pass, for he found that simple healing amongst the wild flowers of the field; and in after years he came to know he did indeed possess the power to heal, and many were the sick folk who were cured by his touch.

His ideal of a simple way to heal all disease persisted, and as he grew older it became a conviction and the activating force behind his whole life's work, for throughout the years he practised as pathologist, bacteriologist and homœopath his one aim was to find pure remedies, a simple form of treatment to replace the complicated scientific means which gave no certainty of cure.

But the boy, Edward Bach, was no mere dreamer. His certainty, his intensity of purpose, his interest in all things, however small, combined to make a character of great genius; though, as is usual with genius, he was destined to stand alone, for few could follow and understand the determination of one who knew his life's work from the start, and would allow nothing to interfere with that great aim.

There were two great interests in his life—overwhelming compassion for all who suffered, whether human being, bird or beast, and love for Nature, for Her trees and plants. These two combined to lead him to the knowledge of the healing that he sought. The one love helped the other, for he found in Nature's storehouse the flowers of the field which heal all those in sickness and in pain.

CHAPTER II

On leaving school at the age of sixteen, Edward Bach, although still determined to enter the medical profession, decided first of all to work in his father's brass foundry, for he felt he could not ask his parents to stand the expense of the long medical training. So for the next three years, from 1903 to 1906, he worked in the Bach factories in Birmingham.

These years, although long and difficult for one of his free, sensitive nature, he considered were not wasted, for there amongst his fellow-workmen he gained an insight and understanding of human nature which was to be the basis of all his future work.

He had no liking for the indoor life and regular hours of the factory, but as was his nature he set himself to learn the work thoroughly, working at the lathes in the workshops, in all the various departments, and trying his hand for a while as commercial traveller for the firm.

In after years he would relate his adventures in this capacity with great good humour. His generous nature and lack of business instincts would not permit him to argue over prices, and he would return from his journeyings with a book full of orders, which the firm, not able to produce the goods at the figures he had agreed upon, could not possibly fulfil. So that he was soon found other work to do.

In 1903 he joined the Worcestershire Yeomanry, where with the horses he was able to indulge his great love of animals; also the open-air life of the camp was an acceptable relief from the noise and confinement of the factory.

But still his chief interest was nature study in all its branches. The trees and plants were to him a world of absorbing interest, and he would rather have worked all night at the factory than lose the daylight for his rambles.

Regular hours were always irksome to him; he knew then that inspiration would come at unexpected moments, and that it was in such moments all real work was done; and so strongly was he guided by inspiration that anything interfering with intuitive action not only gave him a sense of dissatisfaction and unfulfilment, but left him physically exhausted and ill.

This made the three years in the factory seem long indeed to him, and at last he could not resist the urge to begin his true work; and this was strengthened by his knowledge that the fear of ill health was ever present in the minds of his fellow-workmen. To them sickness meant loss of work with the added burden of heavy medical fees, and they would struggle on when often they should have been at home in bed.

He saw also that little was done for the greater number of their complaints beyond palliation and suppression of symptoms, and he determined to find a way to ease their minds and heal their bodies, for he was still convinced there was a simple method of healing to be found, one which would cure all disease, including those called chronic and incurable.

It seemed to him that this form of healing perhaps belonged more to the Church than to the medical profession, for Christ, the Great Healer, healed body, mind and soul; and he debated within himself which profession he should enter.

But neither seemed fully to interpret his ideals, and he began to realise he would need to find out for himself new or perhaps long-forgotten truths about disease and the healing of mankind.

First, he decided, he would study all the known methods of cure, and for this a medical training was necessary, but the question of expense still held him back and he almost relinquished the idea. But when he told his father of his decision and the reason for it, to his great joy his father told him to follow his own bent, and said he would pay the fees and give him an allowance so that he might begin his training straight away.

He lost no time after his talk with his father, but commenced studying for matriculation, and entered as a student at the Birmingham University at the age of twenty.

CHAPTER III

MEDICAL TRAINING

FROM the Birmingham University Edward Bach went to London to finish his training at University College Hospital, where he qualified in 1912.

He obtained the Conjoint Diploma of M.R.C.S., L.R.C.P. in 1912, the degrees of MB., B.S. in 1913, and the Diploma of Public Health (D.P.H. Camb.) in 1914.

From the first day of entering University College Hospital as a student until 1930 he rarely left London. His enthusiasm and intense desire to find the true healing filled his life to the exclusion of all else.

He had no love for city life. The never-ending noise of the traffic, the crowded streets which allowed so little of the sky to be seen, made him yearn for the peace and quiet of the country and the beauty of the trees and plants; and this longing made those years in town at times agony for him.

He would even avoid the London parks, fearing that the call of Nature would prove too strong for him and distract him from his work which, it seemed to him, must for the moment lie where he had the opportunity to study many patients, thinking that only in the hospital wards and laboratories would he find out how truly to relieve the sufferings of those patients. He did not know then that the love of Nature which he was doing his best to stifle was, in the end, to guide him in his search, and that the wild flowers held in their petals a far greater power of healing than any remedy prepared in the laboratory by scientific methods.

Those student years were not easy ones for him in many ways. His diffidence and thought for his father had made him ask for an allowance which was, he

15

found, barely enough to keep him supplied with the books necessary for his studies, and often he was hard put to it to buy enough food to satisfy his hunger by the end of the week. Many were the means he employed to augment his allowance, correcting examination papers and working to all hours of the night to make ends meet. In addition to this his health was not very good and his passion for work gave him little leisure, but his intensity of purpose overcame all physical limitations as it was to do throughout his life.

As a medical student Edward Bach spent little time with his books; even then he felt that theoretical knowledge was not the best equipment for a physician, nor the perfect method of dealing with human beings who differed so greatly in their reactions to the diseases which affected their physical bodies.

To him the true study of disease lay in watching every patient, observing the way in which each one was affected by his complaint, and seeing how these different reactions influenced the course, severity and duration of the disease.

Through his observations he learnt that the same treatment did not always cure the same disease in all patients; for although perhaps five hundred persons, affected by a similar complaint, would react in much the same way, yet there were thousands who reacted in a different manner, and the same remedy which would apparently cure some had no effect upon others.

This caused him to question the giving of particular remedies for definite diseases, and he renewed his study of the patients in the wards, looking for further enlightenment.

Then he realised that patients with a similar personality or temperament would often respond to the same remedy, whereas others of a different type needed other treatment for their cure, although suffering from the same complaint.

Thus early in his search he had gained the knowledge that *the personality of the individual was of even more importance than the body in the treatment of his disease.*

The personality of the patient, the suffering human being, was to Bach the chief indication of the treatment required; the patient's outlook on life, his emotions, his feelings, were all points of first importance in the treatment of the physical disabilities.

Edward Bach spent hours in the wards, watching the patients, longing to find the cure for their ills, instead of temporary relief. He saw how the process of healing was often painful, sometimes almost more painful than the disease itself, and this served to strengthen in him his conviction that true healing should be gentle, painless and benign.

Even in his student days he was beginning to learn much of the truth concerning disease and its cure, and his observations of that time were to become the foundation stone of the new system of medicine he was to discover just twenty years later. Only gradually was he allowed to learn these truths. Step by by step as the years passed he added to his knowledge, making discoveries in every branch of medicine, discarding or perfecting these discoveries as he proved their worth; always with one aim behind all his efforts; the purification of existing medicine and the finding of a simple, certain cure for disease.

Throughout his life he had little use for accepted theories until he had proved them for himself. Practical experience and observation were to him the only true way of learning. Indeed, he was known to have said on being presented with his medical degrees, "It will take me five years to forget all I have been taught."

He gained his knowledge and experience from life and his own intuition, so that the results of his work were all practical; and when finally, at the completion of his life's work, he left the record of it, it was contained in one small book* of thirty pages, written clearly and simply for all to understand.

*The Twelve Healers and Other Remedies, Edward Bach, M.B. B.S. D.P.H.

CHAPTER IV

PATHOLOGIST AND BACTERIOLOGIST

In 1913 Edward Bach held the appointment of Casualty Medical Officer at University College Hospital, and later the same year that of Casualty House Surgeon at the National Temperance Hospital; but he was forced to give up this post after a few months owing to a breakdown in health.

When he recovered he took a consulting-room near Harley Street, where he soon became very busy. As his practice increased he grew more and more dissatisfied with the results of orthodox treatment, for though many of his patients improved, and many were apparently cured, their health was not always maintained. There were many long-standing and chronic cases, too, which seemed to receive no benefit from any form of treatment.

It seemed to him that modern medicine failed in some way, and that surgery could rarely do more than palliate and relieve; and it saddened him, for he could as yet see no way of remedying this. The apparent failure was, he felt, due to the fact that the majority of medical men had little opportunity to study their patients. They were kept too busy to think of the human side, concentrating too much upon the physical body, and so forgetting that each individual was not in any respect built to pattern.

They were taught to be so concerned with disease that they ignored the personality of the human being, and he was convinced that in this way they were neglecting the most important symptoms of the patient.

This made him look around for other methods of healing, and he became interested in another branch of medicine, the Immunity School.

Consequently he became Assistant Bacteriologist at University College Hospital, and hoped, in bacteriology, to find the answer to his problem. From the results of his work he began to feel he was indeed on the track of a method of treatment which would cure even the stubborn chronic cases which hitherto had defied all the efforts of the medical profession, for he discovered that certain intestinal germs, which up to then had been considered of little or no importance, were closely connected with chronic disease and its cure.

These germs were present in the intestines of all persons suspected of suffering from chronic disease, and were also present in healthy individuals; but in the first instance they were definitely increased in number, and in the latter were present in smaller proportion.

His work, therefore, was to study these bacilli and to find out what relationship they bore to the chronic complaints present in patients; why it was they were present in so great numbers, and whether they were there to help or to hinder return to health.

Weeks and months of investigation followed, and as his researches progressed he became convinced that a vaccine made from these intestinal bacteria and injected into the patient's blood stream would have the effect of cleansing the system of the poisons causing the chronic disease. The results he obtained by so doing were beyond all expectations.

Not only did the general health so improve that the patients remarked they had never felt so well before, but the chronic complaint—the arthritis, the rheumatism, the headaches, and so on—disappeared for good.

Though he obtained such encouraging results from these vaccines, Edward Bach disliked the method of injecting them through the skin, with the resultant painful reactions in the patient, and the local pain, swelling and discomfort following the use of the syringe needle; and he set himself to find a simpler method of application.

He partially solved this problem through his next

discovery, for he noticed that if a dose of vaccine was not repeated until the beneficial effects of the former one had worn off, or the patient's condition had become stationary, the results were better than when doses were administered at stated intervals, and there were far less severe reactions in the patient.

This gladdened him, for fewer injections were needed; often weeks, months, even a year would pass before the patient required a second dose, for so long as improvement was maintained no further treatment need be given. Only if there was a relapse or if the condition became stationary need the dose be repeated.

These important discoveries revolutionised the treatment of chronic disease, and a few years later, in another school of medicine—the homœopathic—he continued his researches upon them, improved and simplified them with added success and even better results than before.

His own health at this time was not good, and at the outbreak of the Great War in 1914, much to his sorrow, he was refused again and again for service abroad.

However, there was much for him to do. He was in charge of over four hundred war beds at University College Hospital in addition to his research work in the bacteriological department, and also Demonstrator and Clinical Assistant of Bacteriology to the Hospital Medical School from 1915 to 1919.

He worked unceasingly, giving himself no rest, until he felt so ill that he would faint at the laboratory bench. His great determination not to give in to his own disabilities whilst there was so much to be done and so many needing help kept him going for a time; but in July 1917 he had a severe hæmorrhage and became unconscious.

He was carried into one of the hospital wards and put to bed and his people sent for, for such was his condition that an immediate operation was necessary if his life was to be saved; indeed, the surgeons gravely doubted that they would be in time.

His parents gave their consent, and the operation was performed unknown to Edward Bach, who had never regained consciousness.

He lived through the operation, but still a very grave view was taken; and when he was able to be told he was warned that the disease, although removed locally, was likely to spread; that few recovered permanently from such a complaint; and at the most he would have but three months to live.

Then followed for Edward Bach days and weeks in bed, days and weeks of indescribable pain and agony of body and mind. For one of his active sensitive nature, with the burning urge to live and accomplish his purpose in life, those first weeks were almost beyond bearing. Three months left in which to finish the work he knew was barely begun!

Gradually he became reconciled to the thought, but determined, if he were to leave his work unfinished, he would make as full use as possible of the few weeks of life remaining to him. Still very weak, just able to walk about, he returned to the hospital laboratories, where for some weeks he took entire charge of the department.

At once he became so immersed in his experiments that he lost all count of time, working day and night, until the light shining from his laboratory windows was called "the light that never goes out."

As the weeks and months slipped by he forgot his own disabilities and found himself growing stronger, and when the three months had elapsed he suddenly realised he was in better health than he had been for some years.

The men who had seen him at his worst were astounded at his recovery, so much so that one medical friend who had attended his operation and then left immediately for the front, on meeting him suddenly some time afterwards, exclaimed: "But, good God! Bach, you're dead!"

This made him pause to consider the reason of his marvellous recovery, of his return to life, as it were; and he came to the conclusion that an absorbing interest, a great love, a definite purpose in life was the deciding factor of man's happiness on earth, and was indeed the incentive which had carried him through his difficulties and had helped him in the regaining of his own health.

In his later work this great truth is emphasised, for the herbal remedies he discovered hold the power of so revitalising the mind and body that the wish to live and do one's work in life is regained, and with that desire good health returns.

The vaccines he prepared from the intestinal bacteria were being more and more used in the treatment of chronic disease, and with such excellent results that the method was adopted generally by the medical profession.

During the influenza epidemic of 1918, Edward Bach was allowed unofficially to inoculate the troops in certain home camps with his vaccines, thereby saving many thousands of lives; and he longed to be able to extend this work, for in other camps the death-rate was appalling. He knew he could have prevented untold suffering had he but had the opportunity.

With the return to health, he renewed his researches with increased activity, and his reputation as a bacteriologist brought an ever-growing number of patients to his Harley Street consulting-room.

He was greatly encouraged with the results of his work at this stage, feeling he was gradually nearing the gentler, surer method of treatment he so desired to find. Even now he had been able, to a large extent, to eliminate the need of unpleasant drugs and medicines and, above all, to give hope and comfort to many who had lost all expectations of recovery.

His work in connection with intestinal toxæmia was becoming more and more known, and the results of his findings were published in the medical journals and are recorded in the Proceedings of the Royal Society of Medicine for the year 1920.*

Although these discoveries were a very great advance upon the older methods of treating chronic disease, Bach was still not completely satisfied.

There remained certain diseases which did not respond to treatment, where even vaccines were of no assistance, and the accepted method of diagnosis was, to his mind, far too lengthy. Frequently days, weeks, often months, were spent in investigations, observations and tests before the name of the disease could be decided upon and the treatment prescribed. During this time the patient still suffered and became weaker and more in need of help.

He began to feel his work was as yet in its infancy, and he determined to redouble his efforts.

*"The Nature of Serum Antitrypsin and its Relation to Autolysis and the Formation of Toxins."—F. H. Teale and E. Bach (*Proc. Roy. Soc. Med.* 1920).

"The Relation of the Autotryptic Titre of Blood to Bacteria Infection and Anaphylaxis."—F. H. Teale and E. Bach (*Proc. Roy. Soc. Med.* 1920).

"The fate of 'washed spores' on inoculation into animals, with special reference to the Nature of Bacterial Toxæmia."—F. H. Teale and E. Bach (*Journal of Pathology and Bacteriology*, 1920).

CHAPTER V

HOMŒOPATHY. THE BACH NOSODES

THE latter part of 1918 was to see a new phase of Edward Bach's work.

The authorities of University College Hospital decided that their staff should give all their time to the Hospital and relinquish any outside work they might have. This did not appeal to Edward Bach. His strong dislike of set hours for work, of rules and regulations, caused him to send in his resignation there and then.

But he determined to continue his researches in connection with intestinal toxæmia, and to that end he furnished a small laboratory of his own in Nottingham Place, W.1, where he could both see patients and proceed with his investigations.

He was very hard pressed for money at this time, for he had spent all he had on fitting up his experimental laboratory, and he was forced to live and eat and sleep in one small room; but he was happy, for he was free to continue his researches on his own lines, never doubting that he would gain fresh knowledge and make further discoveries for the benefit of the suffering.

Shortly afterwards the post of pathologist and bacteriologist at the London Homœopathic Hospital became vacant, and on application he was accepted. He began his new work there in March 1919, remaining until 1922.

Then it was he was given the *Organon* to read, the book written by Hahnemann, the founder of homœopathy.

This he started to read with doubt in his mind, but the very first page made him reverse his opinion, for he recognised the great genius of Hahnemann, and he sat up the rest of the night and read the book from cover to cover.

The more he read the more interested he became, for there was a great similarity between Hahnemann's discoveries and his own.

Hahnemann, it seemed, had known nearly one hundred years ago what he had recently discovered for himself by different methods. Hahnemann had found the close relationship between chronic disease and intestinal poisoning; and had also proved that doses were more beneficial if only repeated when the improvement resulting from a former one had ceased.

Edward Bach was profoundly impressed. Here was a man who many years ago had discovered these facts without the aid of modern scientific apparatus; and who, first proving them on himself and his few assistants, had been brave enough to give his knowledge to the world with none to back him up.

The cures which Hahnemann had obtained were doubly marvellous to Edward Bach's mind in that he had used not germs, the products of disease, but remedies culled mainly from Nature, Her plants and herbs and mosses. Poisons and metals had also been employed, it is true, but in minute quantities and prepared in such a way that their harmful effects had been neutralised.

Here was another like himself who had discovered that each case of illness required individual, not mass, treatment. In Hahnemann's words: "Therefore the rational physician will judge every case of illness brought under his care according to its individual characteristics . . . he will treat it according to its individuality . . . with a suitable individual remedy." (*Organon*, para. 48.)

Hahnemann had realised, as he himself had long believed, that the principle of true healing was to *treat the patient and not the disease;* to treat the characteristics, the tempermental side of the patient, the 'mentals' as Hahnemann called them, using these as the guide to the remedy required, irrespective of the physical complaint.

With this method of diagnosis the remedy could be prescribed and the treatment commenced at once, with no loss of time for investigations or long and often painful examinations.

This principle, "treat the patient and not the disease," became the basis of the new system of herbal medicine Edward Bach was to discover not many years later.

He found many of Hahnemann's ideals were identical with his own; the motive which had inspired him from the beginning of his medical career, and was to lead him throughout his life to allow nothing to stop or prevent his carrying out his mission, was expressed by Hahnemann himself in the first paragraph of the *Organon*: "The physician's high and only mission is to restore the sick to health, to cure . . ."

Such an ideal sometimes caused him to be misunderstood and his work questioned by the orthodox, and more than once he was warned that his name might be removed from the Medical Register; but this left him unaffected, for when he was convinced of a better way of healing those in distress he would never conform to accepted rules and theories.

After reading the *Organon* Bach felt that if he could combine Hahnemann's discoveries with his own in some way, he would be able to extend and improve on both.

He had no wish to alter or detract from Hahnemann's work, but he knew that as the times had changed so had the conditions and circumstances surrounding patients, and so indeed had the diseases themselves, for constantly new names, new complaints, were being brought into prominence and, moreover, the class of disease called 'incurable' had been largely neglected.

The work in the bacteriological department of the

London Homœopathic Hospital had long been neglected, and Bach first turned his attention to building it up and overcoming the prejudice amongst the homœopaths against mixing, as they thought, orthodoxy with the pure principles of Hahnemann.

It did not take him long, and soon the work of the department increased to such an extent that he asked for assistants, and was given men who became so interested in their part of the work that he had leisure to begin his own experiments.

He then turned his attention to the relationship between his own discoveries and those of Hahnemann concerning chronic disease.

Several years before his researches in the Immunity School at University College Hospital had led him to discover the fact that poisoning from certain organisms in the intestinal tract was the cause of chronic disease, and that when these toxins were removed the so-called chronic complaint disappeared.

Hahnemann, from his investigations many years before, had realised the same fact. His theory was that there were one or more of three poisons—syphilis, sycosis, psora—which had to be eliminated before a cure of a chronic complaint could be effected.

Although the first two poisons were recognised and definable, as yet little was known of the third—psora—beyond the symptoms present in the affected patient.

Bach came to the conclusion that intestinal toxæmia, the poison set up by certain organisms found in the intestines, was identical with Hahnemann's psora.

He then proceeded to prepare vaccines from these organisms by the homœopathic method of preparation, and gave them to patients by the mouth as medicines, only repeating a dose when the effects of the former one had ceased. The results delighted him, and from that time he rarely gave injections.

He had always disliked the hypodermic needle, and

now he welcomed the better and simpler way of administering vaccines by the mouth, a method which the majority of patients preferred, for not only was the local reaction avoided, but also, in most cases, the general reaction was far less.

These oral vaccines or nosodes, so prepared and administered, fully justified his work; hundreds of so-called chronic cases were treated with excellent results, and he considered he had advanced one more step towards the gentler, better medicine he knew was so needful for the happiness and comfort and quicker recovery of all sick people.

He classified the enormous variety of these organisms present in the intestines into certain groups by means of their fermentation action on sugar, and divided them into seven main groups, which included most of the organisms found.

These seven groups of bacilli he named:

1. Proteus.
2. Dysentery.
3. Morgan.
4. Fæcalis Alkaligenes.
5. Coli Mutabile.
6. Gærtner.
7. No. 7.

The property of the vaccines prepared from these groups he found to be that of purifying the intestinal tract and of cleansing and keeping pure all that was eaten, so that what left the body was wholesome and clean and inoffensive.

This cleansing process resulted in a remarkable improvement in the general health of the patient and cure of the local condition without any local treatment.

Each patient was tested for the bacterial group predominant in the intestine, and either an autogenous or polyvalent nosode given.

By the autogenous method a vaccine was made of the organism isolated from a particular patient, and given by the mouth to that same patient; while, to cover a great number of cases, a polyvalent nosode, one made from collecting organisms from some hundreds of cases and potentising the whole, was administered.

Bach was at the same time working out the 'mentals' or type of personality of the patients in each of whom one of the seven bacterial groups predominated, and he found definite types belonging to each group.

The seven bacterial groups corresponded to seven different and definite human personalities. His enthusiasm was unbounded and he felt he had justified his conviction, for by treating patients according to their temperamental symptoms with these seven nosodes, he obtained results beyond his expectations.

There was a vast amount of research still to be done in connection with the nosodes and the types, and numberless observations and classifications of patients, but as the work progressed he was soon able, to his great joy, to predict to a very large extent from the type of patient and his symptoms alone the organism to be found.

This method of diagnosis appealed to him above all others; patients would be saved the discomfort and embarrassment of physical examinations and investigations which only served to tire and weaken them further.

He was, later on, to develop this method of diagnosing and prescribing to a much fuller degree in the new system of herbal medicine he discovered.

Even at that time he was not at all pleased if he could not recognise the remedy a patient required in the time it took that patient to walk from the consulting room door to his desk.

Increasingly good results were being obtained by his vaccines and nosodes in chronic complaints. The seven oral vaccines, named the Seven Bach Nosodes, were enthusiastically welcomed by the medical profession, and were being widely used not only in England, but even more in America and Germany and many other countries by allopaths and homœopaths.

Bach was untiring in his efforts to make this great benefit to the sick known in all quarters, giving lectures and writing papers for the medical journals.

In his paper, "The Relation of Vaccine Therapy to Homœopathy,"* read to the London Homœopathic Society in April 1920, he pointed out to the homœopaths the resemblance between the most modern branch of science and the teaching of Hahnemann, not only as regards the size of dose, but also in the composition, method of usage and type of remedy. This address aroused tremendous interest amongst the members of that branch of medicine.

During the following years the work of classifying more fully the symptoms peculiar to each particular group of organisms continued. Edward Bach was striving to bring it to such perfection of detail that prescribing would be possible on symptomatology alone, without the aid of the laboratory.

*"The Relation of Vaccine Therapy to Homœopathy," Edward Bach, M.B., B.S., D.P.H.; published in *The British Homœopathic Journal*, April 1920.

CHAPTER VI

1922-1928. THE SEVEN BACH NOSODES (*continued*)

IN 1922 the work of his department at the London Homœopathic Hospital had extended and increased so greatly that Edward Bach had little time for his own researches. His growing fame brought him almost more work than he could cope with at his Harley Street consulting room, and in addition he still retained his small room in Nottingham Place, W.1, where he treated the poor, giving them the benefit of his experience and charging them no fees.

As there was yet a great amount of work to be done in connection with the seven nosodes, he gave up his post of bacteriologist and pathologist to the London Homœopathic Hospital, and shortly afterwards moved to a big laboratory in Park Crescent, Portland Place.

His genius was now generally acknowledged amongst a discriminating circle, and the homœopaths named him the "second Hahnemann."

In 1926 he published his book *Chronic Disease: A Working Hypothesis*, written in collaboration with Dr. C. E. Wheeler of London, who had assisted him in his researches at the London Homœopathic Hospital and afterwards. The book was widely circulated and welcomed by the medical profession, both allopathic and homœopathic, and the results obtained by all who used his methods were so satisfactory that to a large extent the oral vaccines took the place of the injected vaccines.

The next few years were increasingly busy ones. He spent his time between the Harley Street consulting room and the laboratories in Park Crescent. Work poured in upon him so that he had to engage a permanent staff to assist him, but he himself personally prepared the vaccines from specimens sent him by over seven hundred doctors.

In addition to this, medical men from abroad came to work under him in the laboratory for a while to learn his methods, for it was always his wish to broadcast the knowledge of his discoveries so that the greatest number might benefit.

His income at this time was a large one, but every penny he made was spent on the instruments and appliances necessary for his research work, and the salaries of his assistants. He kept so little for himself that when he left London in 1930 to begin his new work he had but a few pounds in his pockets.

Edward Bach was untiring in his efforts to simplify and purify the methods and remedies used in healing; he worked unceasingly all day and most of the night, making further experiments, more discoveries, investigating and testing other methods of scientific healing—electricity, X-ray, the Abrams Box—but never being completely satisfied with the results.

He was at the same time studying the effects of diet in relation to disease, and was advocating uncooked foods, fruits, nuts, cereals, vegetables, to reduce the amount of toxins produced in the intestines.

The effect of this diet, combined with vaccine treatment, was the subject matter of an address he gave to the British Homœopathic Congress, held in London in 1924, in a paper entitled: "Intestinal Toxæmia in its Relation to Cancer," pointing out that "the benefit obtained is due to general improvement and not to local treatment."

Edward Bach was then proving scientifically the principle he had for so long known intuitively—the fact that the patient's temperament was the important indication for the treatment he required. The vaccines so improved the patient's general condition that local complaints disappeared.

Later, with the herbal remedies, he found that "to bring a patient back from 'not quite himself' to 'quite himself' effects the cure."*

At the International Homœopathic Congress in London in 1927 Edward Bach and the doctors who had followed and assisted him in his researches read papers on the work done as far as it had already been proved.†

Dr. C. E. Wheeler of London, in his opening address referring to Dr. Bach's discovery, said: "Its author is going to address you in a few minutes, but I can say for him what he is too modest to say for himself. The fact that I have worked with him for years enables me to speak with knowledge and confidence, and the fact that in the published statement‡ of his theory my name is associated with his shall not prevent my declaring that all I have done has been secondary to his original discovery, and that to him and to him alone belongs the real credit for it.

"Note first that he is a bacteriologist and arrived at his theory by the route of bacteriological investigations —into the problems of immunity, in fact. Note further that, when he worked it out, he knew nothing of homœopathy. His knowledge of this came later and he was readily convinced, and remains convinced, of its value; indeed, he has had no hesitation from the first in making the association of ideas which will presently be formulated for you."

In the address§ given by Dr. Bach himself, he repeated that from his researches and the results of the vaccines

*"The Healing Herbs." Lecture given by Edward Bach at Wallingford, Berks, September 1936.
†"The Problem of Chronic Disease." Addresses read at the International Homœopathic Congress 1927 by C. E. Wheeler, M.D., B.S., B.Sc., Edward Bach, M.B., B.S., D.P.H., and T.M. Dishington, M.B., Ch. B.
‡"Chronic Disease: A Working Hypothesis." Edward Bach and C. E. Wheeler, 1926.
§"The Problem of Chronic Disease."

prepared from intestinal toxæmia, he had come to the conclusion that psora and intestinal toxæmia were identical.

In the last paragraph he said: "The nosode, the remedy prepared from the material of disease, ante-dated bacteriology and the vaccine; but the relation of the latter to the former is obvious.

"To your school, pioneers in the clinical use of disease to cure disease, I offer a remedy which is, I believe, potent against the deepest of all diseases, that chronic toxæmia which the genius of Hahnemann divined and named. If I believe that I can make its nature clearer than was possible for him, I take no jot from his glory —rather I believe I am confirming and extending his work, and so paying him the only homage he would desire."

Dr. T. M. Dishington of Glasgow, in his address,* said: "My experiences have convinced me of the great epoch-making discovery of Dr. Bach's work."

At the same time Edward Bach was making his discovery known to the allopaths who were already using the vaccines extensively. A paper entitled "An Effective Method of Combating Intestinal Toxæmia" was printed in *The Medical World* of March 1928, and another in the same publication in January 1920 ("An Effective Method of Preparing Vaccines for Oral Administration").

In spite of the success of the nosodes and the oral method of administration, he realised that the Seven Bach Nosodes represented only one branch of disease —that included by Hahnemann under the name of psora —and that they did not cure all chronic disease. He was also dissatisfied with the type of remedies used.

It had ever been his wish to replace the products of disease (the intestinal bacteria used as vaccines) by purer remedies, and he determined that his future researches should be to that end.

*ibid.

He set himself to discover the new remedies amongst the plants and herbs of Nature, and he found certain plants which resembled in their effects the groups of bacteria. With these he experimented, but found that there was something lacking which prevented the results from being as good as those obtained by the bacterial nosodes.

In the address* he gave to the British Homœopathic Society in London on November 1st, 1928, he referred to this fact.

That paper, "The Rediscovery of Psora," was published later in the *British Homœopathic Journal* of January 1929, and is of importance, for in it he makes the first public pronouncement of the new and better medicine he was to discover and perfect in a few years' time.

In this connection the following extracts are of great import:

"I wish it were possible that we could present to you seven herbs instead of seven groups of bacteria, because there always seems to be some reluctance in the minds of many to use anything associated with disease in the treatment of pathological conditions."

Referring to Hahnemann in the same address, he said: "He saw that new illnesses might arise owing to altering circumstances of civilisation, and that new remedies would have to be sought. Again his genius comprehended the fact that in Nature might be found an infinite number of remedies to meet all occasions that might arise."

It was in that same year (1928) that Bach found the first three of the thirty-eight herbal remedies which replaced the seven bacterial nosodes. These remedies were to heal any disease and meet all occasions that

---

*"The Rediscovery of Psora." Edward Bach, M.B., B.S., D.P.H. Read to the British Homœopathic Society, November 1st, 1928; published in *The British Homœopathic Journal*, January 1929.

might arise, for, as he eventually discovered, in treating the patient's temperament or mood and not the disease, the kind of illness, its type, name and duration were of no consequence.

In another paragraph he went on to say: "We are making every endeavour to replace the bacterial nosode by means of plants, and have, in fact, matched some of them almost exactly; for example, ornitholgalum in its vibrations is almost identical with the Morgan group, and we have discovered a seaweed which has almost all the properties of the dysentery type; but there is yet one thing lacking, and that one point keeps us checkmated in the effort to avoid using bacterial nosodes. This vital point is polarity.

"The remedies of the meadow and of Nature, when potentised are of positive polarity; whereas those which have been associated with disease are of the reverse type, and at the present time it seems that it is this reversed polarity which is so essential in the results which are being obtained by bacterial nosodes. . . .

"Perhaps at some future date a new form of potentising may be discovered."

It was but two years later that he discovered this new form of potentisation, one by which the difficulty of polarity was entirely removed.

The definition of disease which he gave in the same address* also shows the trend of his new ideas:

"Science is tending to show that life is harmony—a state of being in tune—and that disease is discord or a condition when a part of the whole is not vibrating in unison."

Although the research work upon the oral vaccines was by no means finished, the medical profession was already using them extensively, for Edward Bach, as was his custom, made public his discoveries step by step as they progressed, never keeping back any know-

*ibid.

ledge that might be of immediate use to his colleagues in their fight against disease, saying: "It does not seem right that this benefit should be withheld from humanity."*

He gave freely of his knowledge at all times; fame and reputation made no appeal to him, for his only desire was to restore the sick to health.

*ibid.

CHAPTER VII

1928-1930. THE BEGINNING OF THE NEW WORK AND THE FINDING OF THE FIRST THREE HERBAL REMEDIES

ALTHOUGH most of his discoveries up to that time had been made through scientific research, Edward Bach would trust to his intuition when science could give him no satisfactory answer to his problems, and he found that such inner knowledge always led him aright.

In the new work which he was so rapidly approaching, his intuition, his inspired genius alone was to guide him to truths undiscoverable through the intellect and through science.

The year 1928 was a memorable one, for it was the birth year of the new work.

Every moment he could spare from his practice and work in the laboratory he spent in searching for the plants and herbs with which he hoped to replace the seven bacterial nosodes. He would return from a day in the country or by the sea, after a few hours at Kew or in the parks, with many specimens which he potentised and tested, comparing their results with those of the nosodes, but none of them fully satisfied him.

He pondered deeply upon the reason for this. Being convinced that the true healing agents were to be found amongst the plants and trees of Nature, he sought for a greater understanding of disease itself, its cause and its effect upon mind and body.

Then one evening, dining in a large banqueting hall, he was given the answer to this problem.

Bach had attended the dinner somewhat unwillingly and was not enjoying himself greatly. To pass the time he was idly watching the people around him when suddenly he realised that the whole of humanity consisted of a number of definite groups of types; that every individual in that large hall belonged to one or other of these groups, and he spent the rest of the evening watching all the people he could see: observing how they ate their food, how they smiled and moved their hands and heads, the attitudes of their bodies, the expressions on their faces and, when he was close enough to hear, the tone of voice they used.

So close was the resemblance between certain people that they might have belonged to the same family, although there was no blood relationship.

He found this a most engrossing occupation, and by the time the dinner was over he had worked out a number of groups and was busy in his mind comparing these with his seven bacterial groups. He discovered he had added more type-groups to that number, and knew that when he applied himself seriously to the study he would find even more.

It would be a continuation upon a gigantic scale of the work already done on the nosodes, and he wondered how this extended group-theory would apply to disease and its cure—whether the diseases from which these groups suffered would also bear a resemblance to each other.

Then came the inspiration that the individuals of each group would *not* suffer from the same kinds of diseases, but that all those in any one group would react in the same or nearly the same manner to any type of illness.

He could not wait for the end of the evening's entertainment, but left as soon as he could to think out these new ideas. However, it was not until he had left London in 1930, and was able to give his full attention to the study, that he worked them out in detail.

Every patient who came to him from then onwards was closely observed; every characteristic, every mood, every reaction to disease, each mannerism and little habit was noted and, as far as he was able with the remedies he already had, he prescribed for them on these indications.

The results were so encouraging that he was satisfied his intuition had again led him into the right path. It was the principle of Hahnemann amplified, and it more nearly approached his own ideals of healing than had any method he had practised so far.

One day late in September of that same year he had a sudden urge to go to Wales and, obeying the impulse, he was rewarded by finding two beautiful plants—the pale mauve Impatiens, and the golden-flowered Mimulus —growing in great profusion near a mountain stream.

He brought these back to London and prepared. them in the same way as he had done the oral vaccines. When he came to use them, prescribing them according to the personality of the patient, they had, to his great joy, immediate and remarkable results.

One more plant he found and potentised that year— the wild Clematis, and these three remedies formed the first of the thirty-eight herbs he was to find and use in the new system of herbal medicine he discovered.

With these few remedies he began treating his patients according to their type alone, and an account of them, together with one or two others he had found and used with good results, was published in *The Homœopathic World* of February 1930, entitled "Some New Remedies and their Uses."

So convinced was Edward Bach that he would now be able to replace the bacterial nosodes by the pure and simple herbs of the field that he decided, towards the end of 1929, to give up all other methods of treatment and use these three remedies, the Mimulus, Impatiens and wild Clematis, alone, whilst seeking others to add to their number.

He knew he was on the verge of discovering an entirely new system of medicine, although as yet he had no real conception as to the exact form this new method would take.

So great was the urge to begin the search that he could not rest, nor continue with the work on the nosodes that he and his medical friends had been working hard to complete.

All he had done so far, he considered, was but a step towards this new healing, and he was impatient to begin seriously upon the fresh theories.

At last he told his friends that he was about to give up his work in London and devote himself to the task of finding world-types and searching for the further remedies which would heal these types and, by so doing, heal all the diseases from which they might suffer.

This took his friends by surprise; they had always looked upon him as a leader of scientific research, a genius who had made and would make, further discoveries in that branch of medicine.

They were well content with the oral vaccines; nothing so far had been discovered to compare with them, and they could not follow him in his new ideas which they felt were ideals with but little practical use.

They did their best to dissuade him from going and leaving his work as it were unfinished, but nothing could shake his determination or weaken his conviction that he was on the threshold of far greater discoveries.

Edward Bach's decision to give up all his previous work and begin again was not a light one to make.

His Harley Street practice was bringing him an income of over £5,000 a year; the work of preparing vaccines to send to medical men all over the world was in itself a full-time occupation; and, in addition to this, he was looked upon as an outstanding genius in his own line, with an even bigger future before him.

But none of this did he consider or regret for one moment.

All that concerned him was the certainty which became stronger as the days passed: that his work lay in another direction and that he would find what he sought amongst the trees and plants of Nature; remedies which were already prepared for man by Nature Herself, and were only waiting to be discovered.

He knew, too, that he possessed that divine gift of healing with his hand—the dream of his childhood had come true—for on several occasions during those busy years he had suddenly felt impelled to lay his hand on a patient's arm or shoulder, and that patient had instantly been healed.

Bach never knew when this might happen. He felt, as he would say, a sudden overwhelming compassion, a tremendous desire to relieve the suffering of one who came to him in distress, and he would feel the healing life flow from his hand into the patient, who immediately was well.

Thus, in the spring of 1930, Edward Bach, then forty-three years old, was preparing to begin his work all over again, and on entirely different lines.

His great intellectual powers had led him to make many scientific discoveries, the use of which brought and is still bringing, through orthodox medicine and homœopathy, relief and healing to many sufferers; but now he felt awakening within him that divine inspiration which is intuition, the true wisdom.

Guided by this, he was ready to forsake all scientific and artificial methods of healing and to return to the simple ways of Nature.

CHAPTER VIII

EARLY in 1930 Edward Bach decided to leave London and devote all his time to the new work and the finding of further herbal remedies.

To him decision was instant action, and within a fortnight he had divided his extensive practice amongst his medical friends and closed down his laboratory.

He made a large bonfire of all the pamphlets and papers he had written on his former work, and smashed his syringes and vaccine bottles, throwing their contents down the laboratory sink.

He did nothing by halves.

The work still to be done to complete the method of prescribing the Seven Bach Nosodes he left in the hands of the doctors who had assisted him in the last years. The apparatus of the laboratory and the furniture of his consulting room were quickly sold, and with this money in his pocket, all he possessed, for every penny he had made had been spent on his research work, he left London early one morning in May 1930, after saying good-bye to his friends and, hardest of all to him, the members of the Masonic Lodges to which he belonged.

He set out on his great adventure without one backward thought or regret for the wealth and fame he was leaving, and travelled to the heart of Wales, where he hoped to find and prepare remedies from the simple flowers of the field.

The evening before he left London he was greatly encouraged by the words of one physician, Dr. John H. Clarke, who said to him: "My lad, forget all you have learnt, forget the past and go ahead. You will find what you are seeking, and when you have found it I will welcome you back and give you my support. I

44

have not long to live, but may I live to see the day of
your return, for I know what you find will bring great
joy and comfort to those for whom we, at present, can
do so little. I shall be prepared to give my work to the
flames, and set up instead as a practitioner of the new
and better medicine you will find."

Dr. Clarke lived to hear of the finding of the herbal
remedies called "The Twelve Healers," and before he
died he published the first account of them in his
journal, *The Homœopathic World.*

Now that the time had come for him to say good-bye
to London, Edward Bach was full of excitement and
joy at leaving behind the noise of the traffic, the crowds
and the houses which made him feel shut in and unable
to breathe.

His sensitive temperament had long yearned for the
quiet lanes and fields and woods, and now as he travelled
towards his heart's desire he was as happy as a schoolboy
released from a stuffy classroom.

His enthusiastic nature and tremendous vitality made
him appear far younger than his forty-three years. His
courage—a courage that few possess—was unbounded,
for he started out upon his quest with the knowledge that
he must stand alone, with nothing but his own inner
conviction of great new work to be done to help him
through the years ahead.

Taking a few suitcases with him and the money from
the sale of the laboratory apparatus, he set out with no
plans or knowledge of what might be in store for him,
of what might be the result of his search or, indeed, of
what it was he was seeking, knowing only that he would
find a healing which would be the most practical of all
methods, and which would give results that had never
been known before, for Nature Herself would be the
physician.

On his arrival in Wales he made a discovery which
caused him some disappointment. He found he had

brought with him a suitcase full of shoes in place of the one he had packed with pestles and mortars for the preparation of the new remedies he expected to find.

However, he was soon to be grateful for the mistake. Shortly afterwards he found the new method of preparing the remedies in which pestles and mortars played no part, but the shoes he did need. They became the most valuable part of his equipment, for during the years that followed he walked many hundreds of miles, wandering all over the country, in Wales, the southern and eastern counties of England, by river and sea, watching people and Nature; observing and gaining an understanding of both which led to the finding of the new system of herbal medicine.

Edward Bach had always looked upon healing not as a profession, but as a divine art; and he had grown more and more to feel that those who had the privilege of doing this work of healing should be prepared to give their services, for health was not a commercial commodity, but something which was the right of every individual; therefore from the time he left London to the end of his earthly life he charged no fees for his advice and help either to the rich or to the poor.

Time and again in the years of research which followed he was to suffer great physical hardships and privations through lack of money, but these mattered little to him, nor did they interfere for one moment with his work.

His big-heartedness would never allow him to see others in want, and out of his little he would always find enough to share with them, until it was said of him: "He gave away more than he had."

With contributions from grateful patients and gifts from understanding friends from time to time, he was able to continue his great work; and whenever he contemplated a fresh journey or some new departure in the work, he found he had enough and to spare for all that he might need.

This confirmed him in his belief that he was on the right track, and that all he had to do was to go ahead with complete trust in the Divine Source of all.

CHAPTER IX

MAY-JULY 1930. WALES. THE DISCOVERY OF THE 'SUN METHOD' OF PREPARING THE NEW REMEDIES

EDWARD BACH settled down in a small Welsh village not far from Bettws-y-coed to work out his group-theory and to search for the new remedies.

He had no idea which plants held the medicinal properties he sought beyond the fact that he knew they would all be beneficent and of a very high order, for he was convinced that poisonous substances and plants could have no real function in the healing of the human body.

The right remedies would cause no severe reactions, neither would they be harmful or unpleasant to take; their effect would be gentle and sure, resulting in a healing of both mind and body. He felt also that a new method of preparing these remedies would have to be discovered, a simpler process than those already used.

The springtime of that year came late. The first summer flowers bloomed with their earlier brothers and the woods and meadows, hedgerows and river banks were carpeted with flowers.

Bach spent the day long examining the great variety of plants, noting where they grew, what soil they chose to grow upon, the colour, shape and number of their petals, whether they spread by tuber, root or seed; sitting for hours by a single plant; wading through bogs and marshes, climbing to the mountain-tops, and tramping for miles along the lanes and through the fields in search of fresh specimens, learning all he could of the habits and characteristics of each flower and plant and tree.

Although he was convinced that the plants with the

right medical properties were to be found amongst the simple wild flowers of the countryside, he knew he could eliminate at once the primitive varieties, such as the dodder, the cactus, the seaweeds; and the poisonous plants, the henbane, deadly nightshade, aconite; also the large group of plants used by man as food.

Those which contained true healing power were of a different order and few in number. Many plants possessed medicinal properties which soothed and relieved the sufferings of the human body, and certain of them were already being used in medicine; but the true *healing* plants held a greater power than this.

Their work was not to palliate, but to *cure*; to restore health to mind and body.

As he continued his search day by day, Bach came to the conclusion that these plants would be found later in the year. They would bloom when the days were longest and the sun was at the height of its power and strength; and to obtain their medicinal properties to the full he would need to use the flower-heads alone, for the life of the plant was concentrated in its flower—that held the potential seed.

The plants chosen would be the most perfect of their kind, their bloom beautiful in shape and hue and, as Nature was always lavish in Her gifts to man, they would be found growing in profusion.

One early morning in May as he was walking through a field upon which the dew still lay heavy, the thought flashed into his mind that each dewdrop must contain some of the properties of the plant upon which it rested; for the heat of the sun, acting through the fluid, would serve to draw out these properties until each drop was magnetised with power.

Then Bach realised that if he could obtain the medicinal properties of the plants he was seeking in this way, the resulting remedies would contain the full perfect and uncontaminated power of the plants, and they would heal, surely, as no medical preparations had been known to heal before.

The process of extracting the healing powers of the plants would thus be simple—as simple as the way in which honey, the most perfect of all foods, is collected from the flowers by the bees.

He decided to test his theory by collecting the dew from certain flowers before the sun had caused evaporation, and to try it out upon himself. He first of all shook the drops from various flowering plants into small bottles, filling some with the dew from flowers which had been in full sunlight, and others from those still in the shade.

During his latter years in London, and particularly during the few weeks he had been in Wales, Bach had become aware that all his senses were quickening, becoming more fully developed. He found he was able to feel, to see and to hear things of which he had not been conscious hitherto.

Through his finely developed sense of touch he was able to feel the vibrations and power emitted by any plant he wished to test; and so greatly was his body receptive to these vibrations that it reacted instantaneously.

If he held the petal or bloom of some plant in the palm of his hand or placed it on his tongue, he would feel in his body the effects of the properties within that flower. Some would have a strengthening, vitalising effect on mind and body; others would give him pains, vomitings, fevers, rashes and the like.

He would say that in his laboratory he had had instruments to do the work he was now able to do himself; that he was better equipped than any laboratory, for no scientific appliance could work so well or give such true response as the instruments the Creator had given man in his body—his senses and his intuition.

By these means he was able to test the dew he had collected from the flowers.

None of the flowers contained the healing properties he sought, but he found that the dew from each plant held a definite power of some kind.

The important fact he gathered from this experiment was that the sun's heat was essential to the process of extraction, for the dew collected from plants in shady places was not so potent as that from the plants in full sunlight.

Bach's highly sensitised state was a necessity for the purpose of his present research work, but at times it caused him the most acute distress both of mind and body. Sudden noises, crowds, airless places would utterly exhaust him and leave him in a state of collapse; his face would blanch, his hands tremble and legs shake, and it would often be some hours before he could adjust his delicately attuned senses to the lower, coarser vibrations surrounding him.

This can, perhaps, be better understood by the simile of the highly trained musician suddenly confronted by an orchestra of discords, and the resulting frenzy of jarred nerves.

Only his great courage and intensity of purpose, his extraordinary powers of recuperation and his unquenchable sense of humour carried him through these times of acute distress.

Having proved that the sun-warmed dew absorbed the properties of the plant upon which it rested, he set himself to perfect the new method of preparing the healing remedies.

To collect sufficient dew from individual flowers would be too laborious and take too long a time, so he decided to pick a few blooms from a chosen plant and place them in a glass bowl filled with water from a clear stream, and leave it standing in the field in full sunlight for several hours.

This he did, and to his great satisfaction found the water was impregnated with the power of the plant, and was very potent.

He had now discovered the new method of preparation of medicinal remedies which he had hoped for some years before when he said, in the address he gave to the British Homœopathic Society in 1928 ("The Rediscovery of Psora") "Perhaps at some future date a new form of potentising may be discovered."

The first nineteen of the herbal remedies he was to find later were all prepared in this way.

Bach was overjoyed at the discovery, for this method entailed no destruction or injury to the plants used; the whole process was carried out in the open air in the field where the plant itself grew; the few flowers picked were at their freshest and in the perfection of their bloom, and lost none of their power during transference from the plant to the bowl of water.

It was the method of simplicity he had longed for—the simplicity of mighty things, for fire, earth, air and water—the four elements—were involved and working together to produce healing remedies of great power.

"The earth to nurture the plant, the air from which it feeds, the sun or fire to enable it to impart its power, and water to collect and be enriched with its beneficent magnetic healing," Bach wrote in the paper describing this method of preparation which was published during the latter months of 1930 in *The Homœopathic World* ("Some Fundamental Considerations of Disease and Cure").

This practical and easy method of preparing healing remedies convinced him that true knowledge was to be gained, not through man's intellect, but through his ability to see and accept the natural, simple truths of life.

In the paper referred to above he wrote: "Let not the simplicity of this method deter you from its use, for you will find the further your researches advance, the greater you will realise the simplicity of all Creation."

CHAPTER X

SHORTLY after his first experimental testing of the dew from certain plants, Edward Bach wandered off across the country to study the flora of the coast, finally arriving at Abersoch, the small seaside village a few miles from Pwllheli, and there he stayed until the end of July.

It was at Abersoch he perfected the sun method of extracting the medicinal properties of wild plants and also wrote the manuscript of his book, *Heal Thyself*, the introduction to the new medicine.

The book contains the fruits of the great knowledge of human nature he had gained during his many years of intense study of every type of individual in good and ill health, and explains the true cause of disease and the principles of the new healing.

The manuscript was written day by day as he sat in the fields or sunned himself on the sands after bathing in the sea; and through it runs a great message of hope to all sick people, for he knew that with the finding of the new remedies relief and healing would be brought to many who no longer expected a return of health.

In this book it is made plain that disease of the body is not primarily due to physical causes, but to certain disturbing moods or states of mind which interfere with the normal happiness of the individual; and how these moods, if allowed to continue, lead to a disturbance of the functions of the bodily organs and tissues with resulting ill health, for the mind is in absolute control of the mental and physical conditions of every human being.

Thus any disturbance of the mind, such as continued worry, fear or depression, would not only result in a loss of peace and serenity, but would be communicated to the physical body through the nerves, causing disorganisation of the proper functioning of its organs and loss of tone and vitality in its tissues.

But so soon as the mind regained its normal peace and happiness, it would also regain its wise and perfect control over the body, which would automatically be cleansed of any disease or complaint from which it suffered.

These disturbing moods, then, were the true indications for the treatment of disease; and the function of the remedies of the new pharmacopœia would be to assist the patient to rid himself of the state of mind which was causing his ill health.

The herbal remedies, as Bach wrote in the paper entitled "Some Fundamental Considerations of Disease and Cure,"* would have "the power to elevate our vibrations, and thus draw down spiritual power, which cleanses mind and body, and heals."

In the book *Heal Thyself*, Bach stresses the importance of happiness in life, for not only does it bring health in its train, but it indicates that the individual is living his life on earth to the full, uninfluenced by others; and in so doing, being of the greatest help and service to his fellow-men.

From his own experiences and from watching others closely, Bach realised that man, if he did but know it, was endowed with all the wisdom and knowledge necessary to guide him through his earthly life in the utmost happiness and joy and health; and that this wisdom was imparted to him through his intuition and instincts.

These were the means of communication between man's Higher Self and his earthly personality and, being of divine origin, were to be obeyed and trusted implicitly.

*Published in *The Homœopathic World*, 1930.

Unhesitating obedience to these was the secret of health and of happiness.

When the individual allowed the interference or suggestions of others to deter him from following his own inner convictions, then the conflicting states of mind—fear, indecision, hate and the like—assailed him, marring his happiness and affecting his health.

True happiness, that resulting from "obeying the commands of our soul, our Higher Self, which we learn through instinct and intuition,"* is not only man's birthright, but brings with it all the qualities he strives to attain during his life on earth; the qualities of gentleness, strength, of courage, steadfastness, wisdom, peace and love.

Unhappiness attracts to itself the reverse side of these qualities—greed, cruelty, self-love, instability, ignorance, pride and hate—and these are the underlying causes of disease.

Every man, woman and child is intuitive, although few know the meaning of the word; Bach described it as spontaneity, the ability to be oneself uninfluenced by others. He wrote in a letter to a friend: "What is called intuition is nothing more or less than being natural, and following your own desire absolutely," just like a happy healthy child, never interfering with the happiness of others nor allowing interference, dependent only upon himself.

Bach himself was entirely guided by intuition, not only in his work, but in his personal life. He was always himself, natural and spontaneous, and entirely unaffected by circumstances or other people.

The final paragraph of *Heal Thyself* again emphasises the importance of the happiness which follows man's dependence upon the wisdom of his own divinity, for Bach wrote: "And so come out, my brothers and sisters, into the glorious sunshine of the knowledge of your

*Heal Thyself, Chapter II.

Divinity, and earnestly and steadfastly set to work to join in the Grand Design of being happy and communicating happiness . . ."

When he had completed the manuscript he took it to London and sent it to various publishers, but none of them would publish it on their own responsibility, for they felt it too revolutionary.

Bach had by then come to the end of his financial resources and could not pay for its printing himself. He was very distressed, for, according to his custom, he had wished to make known his discoveries as widely as possible so that all might benefit from them.

This lack of money—from then onwards to the end of his earthly life he had never more than would provide him with bare necessities—would have discouraged all who were not activated by so strong a motive as his; but no hardships or disappointments could deter him from his determination to continue his researches until he had found a more perfect and simple form of healing.

After a few days London became impossible for him; he was still in the highly sensitised state when noise and crowded places exhausted him and made him ill; so he decided to put the manuscript of his book away for a while, and go back to the peace and quiet of the country where he now hoped to find certain of the new remedies, and to prepare them by the sun method of potentisation.

CHAPTER XI

1930. AUGUST. CROMER. THE PRINCIPLES OF THE NEW METHOD OF TREATMENT

FROM London, Bach went straight to the small seaside town of Cromer on the Norfolk coast; there he stayed from August 1930 until the spring of the following year, and during that time he found and prepared most of the twelve remedies which he called "The Twelve Healers," the name by which his sytem of herbal medicine is now known.

He grew to have a great affection for the little town and its people, and although he was to travel in search of plants through many of the counties of England and Wales, during the next four years he returned to Cromer to spend several months each year.

The principles of the new method of healing were now clear in his mind, and he knew his immediate work was to classify the moods or states of mind common to all types of individuals, and to find the remedies corresponding to each of these moods.

"Disease is a kind of consolidation of a mental attitude and it is only necessary to treat the mood of a patient and the disease will disappear," Bach wrote to a colleague at that time.

He had ample opportunity for studying human nature during those summer days at Cromer, for the town was full of visitors enjoying a holiday from work and all the petty worries of their ordinary daily lives; whilst the townspeople were occupied in looking after and amusing the visitors, and the fisherfolk were busy about their own affairs.

Bach welcomed the chance of studying the healthy, normal individual, for he found it gave him an even greater insight and understanding of the difficulties of human nature than the years he had spent in the hospitals amongst the sick.

Every type of individual was represented, and in all stations of life—countrymen and townsmen, fishermen, labourers, tramps, old and young, rich and poor; and he spent much of his time wandering about amongst them on the seashore and in the town, watching them closely, studying their moods and reactions to all the little incidents of the day; and what he saw confirmed the knowledge he had already gained.

Every individual belonged to a definite group or type, having in essentials the same kind of personality, character, temperament as the others of that group.

The members of each group were clearly recognisable by their behaviour, moods or attitude of mind; for instance, the nervous type was fearful of the first plunge into the sea; the hesitating, undecided group took some time to make up their minds to go in; the impatient people walked or ran straight in; the over-concerned tried the temperature of the water first and so on; each individual behaving according to his type.

The same thing would occur in times of sickness.

In an epidemic of influenza each individual would react according to his temperament, showing either fear, indecision, impatience, concern or some such attitude of mind, although the complaint was the same in each case.

The nature of the ailment or disease, therefore, need not be taken seriously into consideration; the *moods* were the indications for the treatment required, for the bodily health was entirely dependent upon the state of the mind.

In the treatment of disease different remedies would be required for each type, each state of mind, irrespective of the bodily complaint.

Bach had realised much of this years before, during his student days in hospital, and had confirmed it in practice later when, as a bacteriologist and homœopath, he had treated patients with autogenous vaccines and nosodes.

He had seen then that all patients of one type would react more or less in the same manner to whatever disease might affect them; that some might suffer from asthma, others from indigestion, rheumatism and the like, but that behind all these diseases would be the underlying cause peculiar to that type.

Then he had believed that this underlying cause was an intestinal poisoning which, when treated and cleared up, resulted in a cure of any complaint from which the patient might be suffering; no local treatment being necessary.

But his recent researches had brought him the conviction that the underlying cause was the moods or states of mind from which the various types could suffer. The remedies he was seeking would assist in the removal of these moods and so effect the cure.

A small worry passing through the mind will cause a look of strain to appear upon the face, so a continued large worry will have a correspondingly greater effect upon the body; but in both cases so soon as the worrying thought had been removed and the peace and happiness of the mind restored, all the ill effects upon the body will go also.

Physical disease, being merely the result of the disorganisation of the function of the brain caused by such moods as worry, fear, shock, strain, was but a symptom itself, and therefore was no indication for the treatment a patient required.

Cure was only obtained through the removal of the cause.

Recognition of the fact that moods and states of mind were alone responsible for ill health would do much to dispel the fear of disease and of the dreaded names given to certain of them, so prevalent amongst both the sick and the healthy. Then, with the patient's co-operation, his earnest desire to get well, there could be no incurable or chronic diseases, for fear of disease is one of the chief obstacles to be overcome in sickness, and the greatest hindrance to recovery.

The property of the new remedies would be that of so revitalising the whole personality that the patient would easily shake off his fears and worries, and with them the disease from which his body suffered.

The remedies used in medicine relieved the physical symptoms of disease, but they did not remove the underlying cause—the mood—and the patient was left without help to rise above his mental troubles. For most this was not easy, and for some almost impossible; hence the long-continued suffering of so many.

In acute disease, the result of violent or quickly passing moods, the disorganising effect upon the body was soon over; but when the mood was not so rapidly dispelled the disorganisation continued, gaining a stronger hold upon the organs and tissues, and the after-effects might become permanent, resulting in 'chronic' disease.

Yet even the so-called chronic and incurable diseases would clear up once the mind and brain regained their normal and wise control of the body.

In some cases the body, owing to long-continued suffering, might be sluggish in its response and gain ground slowly as compared with the mind, but with perseverance it would inevitably respond. The patient's desire to get well was always, however, the deciding factor.

The first and most important sign of progress was the patient's remark, "I feel so much better in myself," or "I feel quite myself again." The restored serenity of mind indicating the arresting of the active disease by the removal of the cause, the disturbing state of mind. The bodily condition would improve and finally clear up with continued treatment.

Edward Bach was progressing far ahead of the ideas of orthodox healing, and he was to go further still, until every method he had previously employed was replaced by a new and simpler one.

As far as his researches had progressed he had reached the conclusion that the health of the body was controlled by the state of the mind, and that the varying moods and feelings were the indications for the remedies required, irrespective of the bodily complaint.

Also, as no two types of individuals were exactly alike in their reactions or moods, they would be affected differently by the same disease and would, therefore, need different remedies for their healing.

Treat the patient's personality and not his disease was the principle of the new system of medicine.

Treat the state of mind or the moods, and with the return to normal, the disease, whatever it might be, would go also.

Moods change from day to day, often from hour to hour, so that the remedies needed, especially in acute conditions, would also have to be changed frequently to deal with each mood as it appeared; thus each time a patient was seen he should be looked upon as a new one who required a fresh diagnosis and a different prescription.

Single remedies or combinations of remedies would be required according to the mood or moods present during the course of the illness.

Threatened illnesses could also be prevented or modified, for the signs of an oncoming disease were clearly shown beforehand by the state of the mind, and treatment in these cases should be commenced when the individual complained of feeling "not quite himself" and out of sorts; then the threatened ailment would not develop.

Although some moods affected certain types of individuals to a greater degree than others, they were at times common to all types.

For instance, fear was very common to the sensitive, highly strung temperament, but on occasions even the most decided and strong-willed individual would feel frightened or even terrified.

Bach therefore concentrated on the moods from which all types and of all ages could suffer, and he found twelve outstanding states of mind:

1. Fear.
2. Terror.
3. Mental torture or worry.
4. Indecision.
5. Indifference or boredom.
6. Doubt or discouragement.
7. Over-concern.
8. Weakness.
9. Self-distrust.
10. Impatience.
11. Over-enthusiasm.
12. Pride or aloofness.

In 1928 Bach had prepared the golden, musk-like flower of the Mimulus Luteus which grows along the banks and edges of clear streams in many parts of England, and had obtained excellent results from its use in patients suffering from a diversity of diseases, but whose outstanding state of mind or mood had been one of fear.

In each case as the underlying cause—the fear—had disappeared, so the physical complaint had cleared up, with a return of the patient's health and well-being.

The account of this remedy, together with three or four others, including the Clematis Vitalba and Impatiens Royaleii, had been published in *The Homœopathic World* of February 1930 ("New Remedies and New Uses").

Clematis, commonly known as the Traveller's Joy, he had given to patients of the indifferent, sleepy type, and the results had been very successful; but this remedy he had prepared from the seeds, and he determined to make a fresh potency from the flowers alone, and so obtain the full medicinal properties of the plant.

The remedy Impatiens, prepared from the pale mauve flowers only, he had given to patients whose outstanding characteristic or mood had been one of impatience and irritability, and the results obtained had been beyond his expectations.

Thus he had already three of the new remedies, and had proved their worth.

He knew there would be certain overlappings and variations of moods which would necessitate further groupings, but he felt that the remedies which would deal with these twelve states of mind would help the greater proportion of sufferers until he had progressed further with his researches.

CHAPTER XII

1930. AUGUST AND SEPTEMBER. THE FINDING AND PREPARING OF SEVEN OF THE NEW REMEDIES

THE results obtained with the three remedies, Mimulus, Impatiens and Clematis, had fully justified Bach's new theory that the indications for the treatment of disease were the varying states of mind or moods and not the physical symptoms of the sufferer.

Not only had the complaints so treated rapidly cleared up, but the general health of the patients had greatly improved, and they had gained an increased happiness and interest in life.

These three remedies thus formed the nucleus of the new pharmacopœia, and Bach had already made them known to the medical profession. The first description of them had been published in *The Homœopathic World* of February 1930, under the title "New Remedies and New Uses."

Although he spent a great deal of his time that August studying the different types amongst the people who crowded the little seaside town, he would often take his stick and tramp the fields and lanes around Cromer from morning until night, searching for the further healing remedies.

He explored the country and its flora for many miles around, from the marshes and river banks of the Norfolk Broads to the salt marshes of Blakeney and Cley further north along the coast; and it was during these wanderings that he came upon seven of the flowering plants he knew to contain the medicinal properties necessary for his new method of treatment.

All of them, with one exception, he found growing by the wayside and in the fields around Cromer. Simple wild flowers which are common to the whole countryside of England.

Some of them had never, so far as he knew, been used before as healing agents; others had been employed as remedies in bygone days, but the knowledge of their powers had been forgotten and they had fallen into disuse. Others, again, were still in use, although their true powers had not been recognised.

The latter remedies were prepared in most cases from the stems, leaves and roots of the plants, which were gathered and often taken long distances to factories, passing through many hands and many processes before they were ready for use. During these many processes the fading, drying plants would, of necessity, lose much of their power.

Bach's method, as has been said, was to pick the flower-heads alone, choosing those which were in the perfection of their bloom, and to extract the medicinal properties from them in the field where the actual mother-plant grew, and in this way none of their life- and health-giving powers were lost.

The first flower he tested for its medicinal properties was the yellow-spired Agrimony, so common a wild flower that many pass it by without noticing its beauty. It grows in abundance on the grassy verges of the country roads and in the fields throughout the English countryside.

Its small blooms are golden with many stamens of the same hue; as the petals fade and fall and the seeds mature, the slender stem is hung with many bell-shaped seed-containers, which are covered with minute hooks. These catch in the clothes of passers-by and in the coats of animals, and so are carried from the mother plant for distribution.

The flower of this plant, Bach found, was the remedy for worry; the restless, tormented state of mind so often hidden behind an outward cheerfulness.

Next he experimented with the strikingly blue flower of the Chicory, then in full bloom amongst the uncut

corn; and he found it was the remedy for those suffering
from over-concern, especially for others. It brought the
calmness and serenity so necessary to those people who
are apt to become agitated and fussy in their care for
others.

A few days later he came upon some plants of the
tiny-flowered Vervain, growing at the foot of an old
stone wall along a cart track, and found it to be the
remedy for the over-enthusiastic and strained state of
mind.

This little plant, which grows about a foot in height,
is so unassuming that it is easily passed unnoticed. The
flowers on its many-branching slender wiry stems are
pale mauve in colour and very small.

Having found these three flowers, the Agrimony,
Chicory and Vervain, Bach potentised them by the
method he had discovered earlier in the year.

He chose a perfect summer day with no clouds in
the sky to obscure the sun's light and heat and, taking
three small plain glass bowls, which he filled with fresh
water, he set them down in the field near where the
flowering plants grew. Then selecting the most perfect
blooms from the Chicory plants nearby, he carefully
picked the flower-heads and placed them in one of
the bowls until the whole surface of the water was
covered.

In the second bowl he floated the little flowering end-
sprays of the Agrimony, and in the third those of the
Vervain.

The bowls were left where they were in the sun for
about four hours until slight signs of petal fading
showed that their medicinal properties had been trans-
mitted to the water. This water, now impregnated with
magnetic power, was crystal clear and full of small
sparkling bubbles.

Bach then removed the Chicory flowers from the
surface of the water, lifting them out with a blade of

grass so that his own fingers should not come into contact with the fluid, for he wished to eliminate the human element as much as possible in the making of the remedies.

The water was then transferred by means of a small-lipped phial to the bottles which were to hold the finished tincture.

When the tincture bottles were half full he added an equal amount of brandy to preserve the fluid and keep it clear indefinitely; and having corked them tightly, he labelled each with the name of the remedy.

After washing his hands to remove any trace of the first remedy before touching the next, he proceeded in the same manner to prepare the finished tincture of the Agrimony and Vervain flowers; afterwards destroying the bowls and lipped phials he had used; for with each fresh tincture he prepared, new bottles and new bowls were employed.

He preferred brandy as a preservative, considering it a purer and more natural agent than the rectified spirit commonly added to medicines.

The next remedy he potentised that year was the flower of the wild Clematis, which grew plentifully near and around the town. Each small Clematis flower was picked just below its head and floated on the surface of the water in the glass bowl, and left in the sun for about four hours; the day again a cloudless sunny one.

The flower of this climbing plant has no petals: it is made up of four to eight sepals surrounding a cluster of stamens, both of a delicate creamy green colour. The plant climbs over the hedges, smothering them with blossom in the summer, and a silver drift of feathery seed-plumes in the autumn.

This, the remedy for the indifferent, sleepy state of mind, Bach had also found to be of great value in cases of fainting and unconsciousness, when, by gently rubbing the gums, behind the ears, the wrists and palms of the hands, return to consciousness had been hastened in a remarkable way.

With the tincture he had prepared in 1928 from the seed of this plant, he had obtained good results in a variety of cases where the patient was of a dreamy, sleepy disposition; but when he came to use the freshly prepared *flower* remedy, the results were even better, and he destroyed the older potency.

Shortly after potentising the Clematis flower, Bach found three more remedies, one of which (the Sow Thistle) he afterwards discarded, replacing it by another.

Of the other two, Centaury and the Ceratostigma Willmottiana, the latter is the only flower amongst the twelve remedies which does not grow wild in England, and is not common even as a cultivated plant. It is a native of Tibet, the land of wisdom.

The Cerato is a shrubby plant, and when in full bloom the mass of deep blue flowers is most striking, almost obscuring the small leaves and the stems tinged with red.

Bach found it growing in the garden of a big house in a neighbouring seaside village, and was so struck by its beauty that he gained permission to pick a few of its blooms. These he potentised at the same time as the little pink flowers of the wild Centaury, whose roots have been used in the healing of disease since the days of old, but whose lovely flowers with their mighty power had so far been ignored.

The Cerato he found to be the remedy for those who suffer from self-distrust, those who lack confidence in themselves; and the Centaury the remedy for those whose outstanding trait is weakness, for it brings increased vitality and strength to mind and body.

By this time the month of September was nearing its end and the days beginning to draw in, whilst the sun had lost much of its power. Bach thought he had little chance of finding further remedies that year, but one day in a field of wheat stubble he discovered a patch of the sturdy little Scleranthus Annuus where the sacks of corn had been dumped for the spring sowing.

The Scleranthus, or Knawel, with its tiny pearl-filmed flowers of green, grows about two or three inches high amongst the roots of the corn. Later it forms seeds which seem almost too heavy and large for its slender stems.

This was the remedy for indecision and all the physical after-effects of that state of mind; and the next fine cloudless day Bach made the potency from the small flower-sprays.

Scleranthus was the last remedy he prepared that year, and he decided to stay in Cromer for the winter months and treat patients with these nine herbal remedies.

CHAPTER XIII

THE WINTER OF 1930. THE PUBLISHING OF THE BOOK
HEAL THYSELF. SOME RESULTS OBTAINED WITH THE
NEW REMEDIES, TAKEN FROM EDWARD BACH'S CASE
BOOK

THROUGHOUT the winter of 1930 Edward Bach was
busy treating patients and making his discoveries
known through a series of articles in *The Homœopathic
World*; also, to his great satisfaction, placing the book
Heal Thyself in the publisher's hands, the first edition
appearing in February 1931.

In the articles published in *The Homœopathic World*
under the title "Some Fundamental Considerations of
Disease and Cure," he described the herbal remedies
and the new system of diagnosing and treatment so far
as his researches had progressed, following his usual
practice of making known immediately any discovery
which would be of benefit to others.

Later he found it necessary to make certain alterations
in the descriptions of the moods or states of mind as
written in those first articles. This was inevitable, since,
as his researches progressed, he gained a fuller and
clearer idea of the different types.

That winter patients came to him in numbers; not
only those living in the locality, but many from long
distances, and he treated them with the herbal remedies,
obtaining results which encouraged him to believe
that when he had found the remaining remedies of
his series of twelve he would have made considerable
progress towards the completion of his work—the
founding of a new and better medicine.

Those who came to him were people suffering from
many and varied complaints, some of which he had in
his earlier professional days been unable to help even
with the aid of science. These, to his immense joy,

either completely recovered or became so much better that life was again worth living for them.

The first patient to whom he gave the remedy Agrimony was an active, restless woman of forty-five; vivacious, always seeking excitement, hiding her very considerable worries and anxieties under a cloak of forced cheerfulness.

Her history was one of alcoholism for many years— mostly spirits. During the last two months the habit had become excessive, and for the last week she had taken practically no food, sleeping but two hours each night. The severe bouts were always associated with worry and anxiety, and when first seen during one of these the patient was semi-conscious, her pupils unequal, pulse 120.

The concealing of personal troubles and worries by external cheerfulness indicated Agrimony, and she was given frequent doses of this remedy. Within thirty minutes of the first dose she fell into a natural sleep lasting three hours. A second dose was then given and seven more hours' sleep obtained.

The second day there was marked improvement; the third day she was about the house, and the fourth day the general condition was better than it had been for months. She continued taking the remedy, and five weeks later was drinking in very strict moderation, the desire for excess having disappeared.

Further doses were given to counteract the effect of serious anxieties and shocks, through all of which she fully maintained the improvement. She became calmer and more restful than she had been for many years. When seen three years later she had still maintained the improvement.

Another patient treated about the same time was a small boy of eight years old, who had been asthmatic from birth. His parents were told that he was likely to suffer from the complaint all his life.

He was an energetic, happy child, full of life and interest, who tried to smile and laugh even during the torment of an attack whilst he was fighting for breath. This again indicated the remedy Agrimony, and for three months he took regular doses of the medicine.

During the first month he had three mild attacks and then no return, and there has been no recurrence since he was treated, now nine years ago.

A man of forty had a severe motor accident seven years before. He fell on the left shoulder, and paralysis of the left trapezius followed and remained. He was unable to raise the left hand above the shoulder, the left scapula was winged and the arm muscles much wasted. He suffered a good deal of pain in the lower cervical region which kept him awake and very restless at night.

He was greatly worried lest he should lose his job, which entailed much active work with both arms, but he concealed his anxiety and the pain he suffered from his family and friends, always seeming cheerful and happy.

In October 1930 he was given Agrimony, which he took for three weeks, and all pain ceased after five days. Within ten days movement began to improve and continued to do so until the middle of December. Further doses of Agrimony were given, and he was soon able to raise his left arm above his head to within two inches of the level of the right arm. There was less winging of the scapula and a great improvement in muscle tone. His general health was very good, and he gained a mental peace and freedom from worry.

These and many other excellent results Bach obtained at that time, proving to him conclusively that the indications for the treatment of disease lay in the mental attitude of the patient alone, and not in the state of his physical health.

In the three cases recorded above each patient

suffered from a different complaint—alcoholism, asthma, paralysis—yet all three required the same remedy, for they were temperamentally alike, cheerful, seemingly happy individuals who made the best of things and tried to hide their worries and sufferings from others.

The indications for the remedy Chicory were clearly shown in the following cases:

A lady, aged seventy, had severe indigestion with pain over the heart. She had had attacks for some years, but worse of late, the cardiac pain and fluttering necessitating rest in bed for one or two weeks at a time.

She was an energetic type, over-concerned about the welfare of her family and household, continually worrying over trifles and never happy unless her children were near her, full of self-pity if they did not come and see her frequently.

She was given Chicory regularly for two months. Improvement began at once and the trouble entirely disappeared at the end of the second month, and when last seen, one year later, she had had no return. She also became calmer and less worried about her family, giving them more freedom and so increasing not only their happiness, but her own.

A lady, aged thirty-eight, in charge of a holiday home for girls, had had catarrh and deafness for one year. The difficulty in hearing was getting worse and interfering with her business capacity. She was very talkative, over-anxious about the welfare of those in her charge, worrying over unnecessary details and always at work.

Chicory was indicated and she took a series of doses in December 1930, marked improvement occurring. In February 1931 she had another series of doses and by the end of the month the deafness and catarrh had completely cleared up. She was also very grateful for the change in herself; she became steadier and quieter, less worried and strained, and in consequence found her work much easier.

Shortly after finding the remedy Vervain, Bach was called to a patient who had slipped on the pavement and badly sprained his ankle. When first seen at 8 o'clock in the evening the ankle was much swollen, stiff and very painful.

The patient was a heavily built man of fifty, extremely impatient, thinking it would mean a three-week's job, which was a serious thing from his professional point of view. His was an enthusiastic nature which caused him to strain and tend to over-work; his strong will kept him going when he should have been at rest.

The impatience indicated the remedy Impatiens, and his tendency to strain and over-work, together with his intense enthusiasm for his work and anything which he might be doing, Vervain.

Two or three drops of each of these remedies were added to a bowl of warm water and a compress of this was placed on the ankle. He was instructed to re-moisten it as soon as it became dry.

The next day he was able to attend to his professional duties, and in the evening was walking normally and was seen stamping his foot on the ground, saying: "I really couldn't have sprained this ankle, after all."

A man of sixty-four had chronic rheumatism in neck and shoulders following influenza five months before. Considerable stiffness and creaking of the neck joints and much pain, which kept him awake at night. He had been subject to attacks of local rheumatism in various joints for several years.

He had devoted many years of his life to church work and the care of the poor and sick. A character of the highest ideals and standards, yet a little rigid in thought and narrow in his outlook.

His attitude of mind indicated Vervain, which he was given for three weeks. There was marked improvement almost immediately, and the condition cleared up by the beginning of the third week. The patient kept free from any signs of rheumatism the entire winter, which was unusual for him.

Amongst those Bach treated with the remedy prepared from the flower of the wild Clematis were patients suffering from asthma, cysts, and the after-effects of sleepy sickness, but in all these cases the patients were of the same type—dreamy, sleepy, disinterested folk.

A woman of forty had been suffering from the after-effects of sleepy sickness for many months, and had been given up as incurable after much treatment. She was dragging herself about her home, tripping and falling down frequently, trying to do a little housework and cooking. She had to sit and rest for long periods, always falling asleep. She had lost interest in everything, her eyes were half closed, her muscles weak and wasted, no appetite.

Her condition indicated Clematis, and within a fortnight of taking the medicine her walking was steadier, she felt less desire for sleep and was able to raise her eyelids and so keep her eyes open for much longer periods.

But the most striking change was in herself. She was happy and hopeful, she laughed and smiled and began to make plans as to what she should do when she was quite well, and was so grateful for her increased activity and strength.

The doses were repeated, and the patient was not seen again for three months, as Bach had gone to the south of England in search of further remedies.

On his return the change in her was remarkable. She was a cheerful, happy woman, doing all her own housework, even the weekly washing, and walking a mile to the town to do her shopping. She also said she had walked to the next village, a distance of six miles there and back, to attend the church, without undue fatigue.

Except for a slight unsteadiness occasionally in her gait she was cured.

A girl of eighteen had had large cysts removed from her thyroid gland six months previously. These were returning and she was told she must wait until they were big enough again, when another operation would be necessary. She was a gentle little girl of the day-dreaming type, very little concerned about her condition.

Clematis given three times a day for a fortnight caused complete absorption of the cysts, and there has since been no sign of recurrence. She was treated in 1932.

Another woman of thirty-six had suffered from asthma all her life. Seven years before she had lost her baby daughter and would still sit for long periods in front of the child's photograph, weeping. She seemed to live in a dream, having little interest in the rest of the family.

This state of mind indicated Clematis, and after two bottles of the remedy she began to regain her joy in life and take an interest in her home. After the first bottle of remedy she had had no more attacks of asthma, and when last seen three years later had had no recurrence.

The latter case confirmed Bach's theory that although many might suffer from the same complaint, yet each might need a different remedy for their cure. This patient suffering from asthma indicated the remedy Clematis, whereas the small asthmatic boy of eight years old he was treating at the same time was improving on the remedy Agrimony. The one was a dreamy, indifferent type, the other a happy, cheerful, alert child, but the physical complaint in both cases was the same.

A typical Cerato case was a lady who had suffered for many years from a distressing and irritating rash which appeared periodically all over her body, neck and head.

Owing to lack of confidence in herself and her own opinions she had deferred too much to the advice of her relations, and in consequence had given up the work for which she had been trained to devote all her time to certain members of her family.

During the attacks when the rash appeared she was almost desperate with the irritation and lack of sleep.

She was given Cerato with immediate results. Within a week she had decided to go back to her own work, and with this determination the rash cleared up. During the seven years since she was first treated she had had slight returns of the rash, but these have quickly yielded to treatment. There has been no recurrence of the very severe bouts to which she had been accustomed.

The remedy Centaury, Bach used that winter in a variety of cases, one of them being a girl of nine years old who had for some months been having attacks of nose-bleeding at intervals of a week, which had necessitated plugging on several occasions.

She was a gentle, quiet child, always over-anxious to please and to do things for others.

The patient was first seen during an attack. She was very bloodless and weak, her state giving rise to anxiety. Centaury was given half-hourly and the bleeding soon ceased. The remedy was continued and the child rapidly regained colour and strength.

A week later there was a slight bleeding which lasted only a few minutes. Since then there has been no trouble and the girl is well and strong. The case was first treated in December 1930, and when seen three years later not only had her physical condition improved, but the difference in her character was very marked. From a weak, suppressed child, imposed upon by her brothers and sisters, she had become full of life and fun, taking her rightful place in the family life.

A boy of twenty-two had been pale and weak and languid for some time, but especially during the last twelve months. His muscles were very relaxed and he was afraid of doing any heavy work because of strain.

There were signs of a small hernia appearing in the groin. Owing to his kind, gentle, willing nature, he was apt to be imposed upon by others.

A fortnight of Centaury, given three times a day, worked wonders for him. Health, strength and colour improved and his muscles became better in tone. The patient had no need of an operation for the hernia, and when seen six months later he was very well and able to hold his own amongst his companions.

A very gentle, quiet child of eleven years old, rather pale and languid, had for a year or two appeared to be getting frail and tired, and had no energy for games. Her parents tried ordinary tonics for some time without success; she did not respond to treatment.

Centaury was given for a period of five weeks, and at the end of that time the child had recovered colour and vitality, and was stronger than she had been for some years.

Scleranthus, the remedy for indecision, Bach gave, almost immediately after finding and preparing it, to a fisherman who had had attacks of severe gastric pain and vomiting each autumn for several years. He had been confined to his house or bed whilst the attacks lasted for about two months each year.

The patient was typical Scleranthus, full of indecision; his condition also varied much from day to day. He was first seen at the beginning of October 1930, when the annual attack had just started and got a firm hold. The patient was confined to the house.

Scleranthus was given hourly and in five days' time, to the surprise of everybody, he was out in the life-boat and then resumed fishing, neither of which he had been able to do for some years at this period.

Doses were continued for three weeks, although the recovery had been complete. In the autumn of 1931 there was no return. In 1932 there were slight symptoms which one single dose of Scleranthus completely corrected.

A professional man of about fifty-five had not been well for some years with periodic attacks of nervous and gastric trouble. He was of the type tortured by the inability to know his own mind and to make decisions. Physically his gait was jerky and unsteady.

Finally he grew into a state of desperation and had the poison before him to commit suicide, but even in this was unable to make up his mind as to whether poison or drowning would be better. Fortunately he was seen by Bach whilst pacing about at this stage.

Scleranthus was given every few minutes and the patient watched for two hours, by which time he had become much steadier and calmer. The remedy was continued for some days, and since that time there has been no need to repeat the dose. The patient has remained in good health a period of two years and his character has become much more positive.

CHAPTER XIV

1931-1932. THE FINDING AND PREPARING OF THE LAST THREE REMEDIES OF THE *TWELVE HEALERS* SERIES. THE WRITING OF THE BOOK *FREE THYSELF*

As the winter drew to a close and the spring of 1931 approached, Edward Bach grew restless; he felt he must be free of patients for a while in order to devote all his time to the search for the few remaining remedies to complete his series of twelve. One day near the end of March he suddenly decided to go back to Wales, and he left Cromer that morning.

Although the winter had been a busy one he had charged his patients no fees, and as usual started off on his wanderings with very little money in his pockets. But this worried him not at all, for he had learnt from experience that help would always be sent him through some agency when it was most needed to enable him to continue his work. This had occurred so often; the last time had been a few weeks before he left Cromer.

When he decided to give up his work in London the previous spring he had had an income-tax deficit of £400; he had gradually paid off £390 of this with the money coming to him from certain outstanding accounts from his former London patients; now he was being pressed for the final £10, which he could not pay. He was wondering whether the sale of his few remaining clothes would bring him in enough when he received a cheque for the exact amount from a patient he had treated and cured in London many years before, and who had not been able to settle up with him at the time. The letter had been weeks in transit, as the patient lived abroad and Bach had had numerous changes of address, but it arrived on the very day for him to settle his debt.

In Wales he spent long days wandering over the

mountains, speaking only to the shepherds he met, pondering on the work he had still to do and the remedies still to find.

He saw clearly the whole scheme of his future work and realised that the road before him would not be an easy one. The new system of medicine, the new knowledge he had gained, was revolutionary according to the ordinary accepted standards, and he would have great difficulty in convincing the majority of people of its truth, would even rouse resistance and antagonism in many.

The great proof of the value of his discoveries would be in the results. This proof he had already obtained in the cases of patients who had been cured with the herbal remedies of complaints which had seemed hopeless, of diseases which had persisted for years in spite of the many treatments tried.

When the time came for him to leave Wales he found he had not enough money for his train fare back to London, but, as usually happened to him, within two days a letter came from a grateful patient enclosing enough for his needs, and he made his way down to Sussex, where almost immediately he came upon the Water Violet growing in the dykes near Lewes. It was growing in profusion, the spreading, fern-like leaves lifting the slender stems and pale mauve flowers well above the surface of the water, and he knew it to be one of the remedies he was seeking.

He extracted the medicinal properties from the flowers by the sun method of preparation, and proved it to be the remedy for the quiet, aloof individuals who prefer to be alone in their sufferings and bear their troubles in silence.

From Sussex he wandered on to the Thames valley, where he stayed for some weeks in a riverside village a few miles from Wallingford in Berkshire, studying the water plants, spending long sunny days in a punt, tramping over the Chiltern Hills and along the country lanes.

He knew, from the extraordinary inner knowledge he possessed, that one of the remaining remedies he sought would be contained in the flower of the autumn Gentian, and that this would be the remedy for the doubting state of mind in those who become too easily discouraged and depressed.

It was then July and too early for the flower, although he found the plant in leaf on the hills beyond the village of Eweleme in Oxfordshire and, hoping to find it at Cromer, where so many of the remedies had been prepared, he returned there to search the countryside for miles around, but without success. It was not until late September that he came upon the plant in flower on a hillside close to the winding Pilgrims' Way in Kent, and he immediately prepared the tincture from the blooms.

Bach had now eleven of the twelve remedies, but as the summer was nearly over he knew he would not be able to find the twelfth that year, and he returned to Cromer again for the winter, where he spent busy months treating patients and gaining increasingly good results with the remedies.

With the return of spring in 1932 his restlessness also returned, and as his many friends and patients had never ceased asking him to come back to London and practise there again, he decided to see whether he could stand the town for a few months until the time came to go in search of the last remedy to complete the series of twelve.

He took a consulting room in Wimpole Street, where he would soon have become overwhelmed with work, but he found the lack of air and space in the town too much for him. The noise and crowds affected his sensitive state of mind and body so greatly that he suffered intensely, becoming ill and tortured both mentally and physically.

Only in the comparative quiet and peace of the parks could he find relief, and he would sit for hours under the trees in Regent's Park until his mind and body regained vitality and strength.

During those hours in Regent's Park a little book, *Free Thyself*, was written, which explained in a simple and practical way how man could learn to follow his intuition; and how, by trusting that inner knowledge, he would be guided in every detail of his earthly life, making it one of health and happiness and usefulness. Included in the book was a description of the remedies he had found and their uses.

The little book was printed in pamphlet form that same autumn of 1932, but when it was sold out he had no further copies made, for he had found more remedies and had written the book *The Twelve Healers*.

After two months in London he felt he could not stand the strain any longer, and he was impatient to find the last remedy of the series, so he travelled down to Kent to recover his strength in the space and freedom of the country

This last remedy he knew to be one of the most important. It was the one to combat the state of terror in those in danger or acute distress. An incident which had occurred shortly before he left London had impressed upon him the great need of such a remedy.

He had been called to a patient who had had a sudden hæmorrhage and was in a serious condition. When seen she was in a very exhausted state, and still vomiting blood. She and those around her were terrified, not knowing what to do.

Bach went to her, and putting his hand on her shoulder, said: "Why, what is this? You will soon be well. Lie down and go to sleep." The bleeding had instantly ceased and she had slept for three hours. On waking she had eaten and smoked a cigarette, and in the afternoon had walked out of doors.

In cases such as this, when things were desperate, in times of panic and emergency, the terror remedy would be invaluable.

Bach's power of instantaneous healing was personal to him; he longed to be able to show others that they could also possess the same powers, but at that time he did not know the way. He could, however, find and give them a material agent, a herbal remedy which would act in the same manner.

Tramping about the country near Westerham, in Kent, he wandered back to the field where he had found the autumn Gentian the previous year. Now the ground was carpeted with the golden blooms of the little wild Rock Rose, and he knew it to be the remedy for terror, for he was guided by the same inner knowledge which inspires the musician to write his melodies and the poet his verses.

The tincture from the flower of the Rock Rose completed the series of remedies which he named "The Twelve Healers," and he returned to Cromer for the winter months, where he gained increased confirmation of the value of his method of treatment in the excellent results obtained.

CHAPTER XV

WINTER 1932. CROMER. THE CORRESPONDENCE
WITH THE GENERAL MEDICAL COUNCIL. REPORTS
OF CASES TREATED WITH THE THREE REMEDIES:
WATER VIOLET, ROCK ROSE AND GENTIAN

As the medical profession was slow in accepting the
new ideas of healing and of using remedies of such
simplicity, Bach decided to spread the knowledge of
his method of treatment amongst the lay people, the
sufferers themselves, and to describe the remedies and
their uses in so practical and simple a way that even
those with no knowledge of the human body or of the
theory of disease could understand.

He began by writing articles for the newspapers and
various magazines, but had difficulty in getting them
accepted; then he finally made up his mind to put a
short advertisement in the bigger daily papers, hoping
in that way to bring the herbal remedies to the notice
of a few readers. He was aware that this method might
lead to his name being removed from the Register of
the General Medical Council, but that was of little
consequence to him so long as he could make his discoveries known for the benefit of the sick.

In due course the advertisement was sent off to four
daily papers; two of them returned it, asking him if he
realised it might cause him trouble with the General
Medical Council, but two others published it, and he
had numerous letters from people enquiring for more
details.

Shortly after the appearance of the advertisement the
General Medical Council wrote asking him for an
explanation, and the following correspondence passed
between them.

26th November, 1932.

DEAR SIR,

My attention has been drawn to the following advertisement which appeared in the *Northern Daily Telegraph* of November 24th, 1932:

'Heal Thyself.' There are British herbs of great value within the reach of all. Information gladly given. Dr. Bach, M.B., B.S., D.P.H., B . . ., P . . . L. . ., A . . ., S . . .

I shall be glad to know whether this was inserted with your knowledge and consent. I enclose a form in case you desire to notify a change of address.

Yours faithfully,

—— Registrar.

In reply to this Bach wrote stating he did not wish to notify any change of address, whereupon he received the next letter on November 30th, 1932:

DEAR SIR,

I have received your letter of the 29th of November. I enclose a copy of the Council's Warning Notice in regard to advertising for the purpose of procuring patients, and I shall be glad to know if you have any observations to address to me in regard to your action, which appears to be a contravention of this Warning and therefore to render you liable to further action on the part of the Council.

Yours faithfully,

—— Registrar.

Bach's reply was brief:

December 2nd, 1932.

DEAR SIR,

The advertisement was for the public good, which, I take it, is the work of our profession.

Yours truly,

EDWARD BACH.

3rd December, 1932.

DEAR SIR

I have received your letter of the 2nd of December, and I shall be glad to know whether you intend to continue to advertise in the Press, or whether the notice to which I have drawn your attention was an isolated instance.

Yours faithfully,

—— Registrar.

To this letter Bach made no reply, and he received a further reminder a week later:

9th December, 1932.

DEAR SIR,

I find that I have had no reply from you to my letter of the 3rd of December asking whether you intended to continue to advertise in the Press, and I shall be glad if you will kindly give the matter your attention and let me have a reply.

Yours faithfully,

—— Registrar.

December 12th, 1932.

DEAR SIR,

I am merely endeavouring to bring to the notice of the British public certain herbs which have healing properties, are harmless, and can be used by anyone.

The report of these herbs has been published in medical papers and brought before the profession. If I feel that certain articles in the Press or further advertisements are necessary, I shall be compelled to use these methods.

Yours truly,

EDWARD BACH.

13 December, 1932.

DEAR SIR,

I have to acknowledge your letter of the 12th of December, which shall be brought before the authorities of the Council in due course.

Yours faithfully,

—— Registrar.

For some months there was no further correspondence until, on April 11th, 1933, Bach received the following letter:

DEAR SIR,

My correspondence with you in November last in regard to your announcement in the *Northern Daily Telegraph* of November 24th, 1932, was brought before the Penal Cases Committee of the Council at their meeting on the 10th instant.

I was directed to say that you should carefully consider the Council's Warning Notice in regard to advertising, a copy of which has already been sent to you, because, if it were contravened, you would render yourself liable to be summoned to appear before the Council in answer to a charge.

Yours faithfully,

—— Registrar.

Bach made no reply to this and forgot all about the matter until the following November, when he again received a letter from the General Medical Council:

2nd November, 1933.

SIR,

I am directed by the President of the Council to inform you that the attention of the authorities of the Council has been drawn to your failure to reply to the Registrar's letter of the 11th April, 1933, sent to you on behalf of the Penal Cases Committee of the Council.

I am accordingly to repeat the warning conveyed to you by that letter, namely, that you should carefully consider paragraph 6 (*a*) of the Warning Notice issued by the Council, which relates to advertising by registered medical practitioners, since any contravention of its terms would render you liable to be summoned to appear before the Council in answer to a charge.

A further copy of the Warning Notice is enclosed herewith, together with a copy of section 14 of the Medical Act, 1858.

In pursuance of that section I am to enquire whether you have ceased to practise, or have changed your residence; and to say that if no answer is returned to this letter within the period enacted by the section, your name will be erased from the Medical Register.

> I am, Sir,
> Your obedient Servant,
> —— Registrar.

November 4th, 1933.

DEAR SIR,

In reply to your letter of November 2nd. I desire to state that I have not ceased to practise, nor do I wish any change in my present address, B . . ., P . . . L . . ., A . . ., S . . ., which was registered during correspondence with Mr. —— in a letter of November 28th, 1932.

> Yours truly,
> EDWARD BACH.

That was the close of the correspondence, and Bach had no further communications from the General Medical Council until 1936, three years later.

Edward Bach was fearless in all things, especially when any limitations or restrictions were likely to be enforced in connection with his work. When he was convinced of the value of a discovery that would be of benefit to the sick, he would let nothing stand in his way; no loss of personal status, no discouragement, no disbelief on the part of others could stop his employing all the means in his power to make the discovery known.

The winter of 1932 brought him many patients, all of whom he treated with the twelve herbal remedies alone, using either single remedies or combinations of remedies as indicated by the moods or states of mind present.

With Rock Rose, Water Violet and Gentian, the three remedies he had found that year, he obtained immediate and excellent results, as the reports of the few cases below clearly show.

A lady about forty years old had had vague pains in the abdomen for three weeks, and rapid swelling of the glands in the groin, axillæ and neck. On examination there were large masses in the abdomen, and the blood count was that of an acute leukæmia. The outlook, of course, was extremely serious.

The patient realised that she had a malignant disease, was in terror and secretly thinking of the easiest way to commit suicide.

The extreme seriousness of the complaint and the patient's terror indicated the remedy Rock Rose, which was given for ten days with lessening of the abdominal pain and a diminution in the size of the glands.

The patient's attitude then changed; she was encouraged by the improvement and the black dread and terror of death had passed away. There was now a quiet fear that the improvement was too good to be true, hence Mimulus was given for about two weeks. At the end of that time the patient's condition was normal, and she has remained perfectly well since she was treated in 1932, a period of four years.

A boy aged eight years had run a thorn into the big toe of his left foot. A small abscess formed and quickly healed. One week later, a Sunday, a painful swollen gland appeared in the groin, the child was not feeling well, and the doctor called in ordered bed and fomentations.

The following Wednesday the child suddenly became worse. The doctor was again sent for and ordered hospital and operation, but the father refused to allow the child to go to hospital. The doctor said it was too serious to operate upon at home.

The child was first seen by Edward Bach on the Wednesday at 8 p.m. There was a lump in the groin three inches in diameter; the skin over this was bluish-red, and the child obviously ill with temperature and rapid pulse, the eyes sunken. The case looked dangerous.

The child was very restless, also fretful and wanting his mother with him all the time, and the case was one of urgency, hence the following three remedies were given: Agrimony for the restlessness; Chicory for the fretfulness and desire for attention; and Rock Rose for the urgency. They were administered half-hourly.

At 10 p.m. the child became delirious. The doses were continued, and by 3 a.m. he fell into a sleep for four hours.

Next morning, Thursday, there was some improvement in the general condition, and the swelling was not quite so tender or so red. Owing to the delirium of the night before, Clematis was added to the other three remedies and continued throughout the day.

Thursday evening, general improvement and a ten-hour peaceful sleep during the night. Friday morning, marked improvement, generally and locally.

All urgency and the fretfulness had gone, so Rock Rose and Chicory were stopped. The child was still restless, obviously weak and despondent, so the remedy Agrimony was still continued; Centaury added for the weakness, and Gentian for the despondency.

Saturday morning, the child almost normal, still a little restless and some weakness; therefore Agrimony and Centaury were continued.

Sunday, the child out of doors all day; and Monday, on the sands, running about, flying a kite.

A man of thirty-eight had severe rheumatism for five weeks. When first seen every joint in his body was affected with swelling and tenderness; he was in great pain, rolling about in his torture, unable to keep still.

Agrimony was given hourly for twenty hours, when there was marked improvement; the pain and swelling had all gone except in one shoulder joint. The patient was calmer and less worried. Agrimony was continued for another six hours, when the patient slept for four hours. On waking all pain had gone.

The next stage was one of fear; fear of the pain coming back, fear of moving in case it caused a recurrence. Mimulus was given for these indications, and the next day the patient was up and dressed and had shaved himself.

But in spite of the good result, the patient felt depressed, discouraged and downhearted. Gentian was given for this mood, and on the third day from the first dose of Agrimony the patient was out and about. He attended the cinema and also visited the local tavern.

A lady had acute rheumatism for two years, and had been either in nursing homes or hospitals the whole of that time. When first seen the hands were very stiff and painful, the ankles double their normal size, and the patient only just able to walk. In addition there was pain in the shoulders, neck and back.

The lady was one of exquisite gentleness, calmness and courage, and had borne her illness with wonderful patience and fortitude. Water Violet was clearly indicated, and was given for two weeks, definite improvement occurring.

At the end of four weeks the patient was able to walk two miles, but felt unsteady and uncertain. The remedy Scleranthus was then given for a few days. Then followed a period of a little impatience and wanting to be back and doing everything for herself, which indicated Impatiens.

At the end of eight weeks the patient had walked four miles, could use her hands freely, had no pain and, with the exception of a little stiffness and a trace of swelling in the right ankle, was completely cured.

CHAPTER XVI

Now that he had found the remedies to correspond with the twelve main groups or types of individuals, and had proved their worth, Bach began to think about the next series of remedies, and he decided he must leave Cromer and the patients who occupied so much of his time, and go elsewhere in order to be free from interruption to carry on his research work.

He left Cromer in January 1933, going first to Eastbourne and then to Marlow on the Thames, where he stayed for several weeks.

Here, at first, he was able to concentrate on the types and states of mind for which the next remedies were required, for he had left no address to which letters might be sent, and as yet no one had discovered his whereabouts.

The next remedies, he knew, would be for the states of mind which had become more persistent than those of the first group. They would be for the people who had grown to believe that nothing more could be done for them, and either became hopeless or struggled on, thinking they must put up with their disabilities and adapting their lives and their natures accordingly, until they had partially or entirely lost their own individuality. For those who had been ill for so long that the irritability, the hopelessness or the over-concern had grown almost part of their natures.

The remedies to help such states of mind Bach felt must be powerful indeed, and would be found in the flowers of those plants and bushes and trees which grow together in masses or great clumps, and which strike the eye by reason of their blaze of colour, beauty and grandeur. The massed power contained in those plants and trees would give remedies containing the necessary stimulus to lift the sufferers out of the groove or rut or the state of resignation to which they had grown accustomed.

Bach soon found the first remedy of this new series in the flower of the Gorse bush, which grows abundantly and in masses on commons and hillsides, the myriad golden blooms filling the air with an almost over-powering scent in the spring and early summer; and he extracted the medicinal properties by the sun method of preparation. He picked flowers from the bushes around the circumference of the gorse patch and from here and there within, collecting in this manner the power of the mass.

Gorse he found to be the remedy for those who had been ill for so long that they had grown hopeless of recovery, and had ceased their efforts to get well; only under persuasion seeking further help.

The remedy had been prepared just before Easter, and from then onwards Bach had little leisure for further research. His whereabouts had been discovered and patients wrote to him and came to see him in numbers. But in the intervals of seeing patients and dealing with his heavy correspondence, he wrote the manuscript of *The Twelve Healers*, in which he described the first remedies he had found, the moods or states of mind they relieved, and full instructions as to preparation, prescription and dosage.

The manuscript was printed locally in pamphlet form, and he decided to sell it at twopence a copy in order that all could afford to buy it and benefit from the herbal remedies. He hoped in this way to cover the cost of printing the pamphlet, for, as usual, he had little money to spare; but this he never did: he would send copies to all who asked for them, always forgetting to ask for two pennies in exchange.

The next remedy of the new series he had found to be the minute female flowers of the oak tree, which contain the medicinal properties necessary to help that type of temperament which struggles on in spite of difficulties, never losing hope or ceasing to make efforts—the opposite state to that of the Gorse type, who becomes hopeless and gives up the struggle.

He decided to prepare this remedy from the oak trees growing around Cromer, and returned there in April 1933 to stay in the town until February of the following year.

During that time he found and prepared the other remedies to complete the further series of four which he named 'The Four Helpers.'

The Oak blossom was potentised in May by the sun method; the flowers were picked from the large group of trees growing round the site of the ancient Roman camp at Felbrigg, near Cromer.

It was not until the autumn of that year that he found the last two remedies of that series, Heather and Rock Water. The intervening months he spent treating patients and further proving the value of the herbal remedies, also working out the indications for the remaining two.

By this time many people, both in England and abroad, were using the Bach herbal remedies and with excellent results, and Bach felt he had been justified in placing the knowledge of his discoveries in the hands of the lay people as well as making them known to the medical profession.

The very simplicity of the method of treatment, the harmlessness of the remedies combined with their great healing properties, appealed to the many who had suffered for so long and had spent so much of their time and money vainly seeking relief.

In order that the herbal remedies should be available and within the reach of everyone, Bach had presented complete sets of the mother tinctures to two big London chemists, asking no return for the gift, but urging them to sell the remedies to the public as inexpensively as possible.

The next remedy he sought was for those people who dislike being alone and are only happy when surrounded by others; they like to talk much and discuss their ailments and affairs with anyone who happens to be near.

One day he asked someone in whom these characteristics were well marked which tree or plant in Nature most appealed to her, and unhesitatingly came the answer: "When I see the heather in full bloom it almost makes me gasp. I forget myself and can only stand and stare."

Bach tested the Heather flower for its properties and found the plant held the power to help that type of individual, so he paid a flying visit to Wales, where, near to the spot he had found the first two remedies, Mimulus and Impatiens, he prepared the Heather by the sun method of potentisation.

At the same time he also prepared the fourth remedy, Rock Water, taking it from an old, forgotten well, which had in days gone by been renowned for its healing properties.

This last remedy he proved to be for those people whose rigid ideals and principles lead them to restrict and deny themselves of much which is really necessary for their health and well-being.

With the tinctures of these two remedies he returned to Cromer, and immediately used them with excellent results upon patients who had as yet gained little benefit from treatment.

A lady of thirty years of age had suffered from asthma for many years, and when seen was just recovering from a nervous breakdown.

She was depressed and had lost hope of cure, both for

her asthma and her general condition, and was very afraid she would not be able to work and earn her living, which was necessary for her.

The hopelessness indicated Gorse, and the fear of loss of work the remedy Mimulus. She had the first bottle of medicine on April 22nd, 1933, and within a few days there was some slight improvement in her general health and spirits. The same remedies were again given on May 15th with added improvement. She felt equal to returning to work, was sleeping and eating better, also the breathing was easier; she had had no further severe attacks.

Her condition varied from day to day: one day she felt much better, the next would relapse into hopelessness and lose interest in her work; thus on May 25th she was given Gorse, Scleranthus and Clematis for these indications. Scleranthus for the lack of stability, and Clematis for the loss of interest. This prescription was repeated until the end of June, when she felt very well and had had no attacks of asthma for the last six weeks.

In December of that same year she had another attack of asthma and was given a further bottle of medicine. Her general condition had been good and she had been at work the whole time.

A young woman of twenty-two suffered from painful and tired feet, for which she could get no relief. Her occupation was one which entailed much standing and walking about the house. She was very depressed and hopeless, as nothing seemed to ease the pain. She had no joy in life and did her work without interest.

She was given Gorse and Clematis as medicine, and a lotion of the same remedies to bathe her feet, which gave her relief within a few days. She was given a further supply of the same remedies, which completely cleared up the painful condition, and she had no return.

A man of forty years of age had an unpleasant-looking wart on the forehead which caused him much discomfort. He was of a jovial type, most happy when surrounded by companions to whom he could talk, apt to speak much about his own affairs and health. This state of mind indicated Heather, which he was given as a lotion. Within three weeks of the first application the wart had entirely disappeared, leaving no scar or trace upon the skin.

A middle-aged lady was subject to profound fits of depression which affected her general health. She slept badly, had no appetite and was rapidly losing weight. She made every effort to get well, struggling against the apathy and depression, trying to forget her difficulties in her work. She was inclined to be strict with herself, allowing herself few pleasures, having very rigid ideals and principles.

Her efforts to get well and the struggle she made to overcome her difficulties indicated the remedy Oak; the apathy and loss of interest during the bouts of depression, Clematis; the fixed ideas and determination, Rock Water.

She was delighted with the results of the first bottle of these remedies. The bouts of depression were fewer and more easily shaken off, she was feeling stronger physically, eating and sleeping better.

The prescription was repeated three times during the following two months, and at the end of that time she considered herself cured. She was cheerful and interested in her work, eating and sleeping normally, and began to enjoy simple pleasures which she had denied herself hitherto.

An elderly lady had suffered for some long time from a tubercular condition of both hip joints. Little hope was given her of relief, and she had been told that she must make no attempt to sit up in bed, as it would lead to serious consequences and great pain.

She was of a cheerful disposition, making light of the very great suffering she endured; but being of an active, restless temperament, she felt impatient of her helplessness and inactivity.

The cheerful hiding of her pain and bodily torment indicated Agrimony, and the impatience, the remedy Impatiens; these two remedies were first taken early in May 1933.

After a few doses the great pain lessened, and within the next three weeks, during which she persevered with frequent doses of the same two remedies, the pain had entirely gone. She began to feel stronger, the relief from pain allowing her to sleep and rest.

Then she had a slight relapse and the pain returned; this caused her to lose heart and she felt hopeless of any permanent benefit. This hopeless state of mind indicated Gorse, which she took for two weeks, when improvement again occurred; the pain ceased and she felt she was strong enough to sit up in bed, which she did for an increasing period of time each day.

She was so encouraged and overjoyed at the progress that she made every effort to get well, and struggled against any thought of depression or doubt. The remedy Oak was then given and she took it as a medicine for three months until, in August 1933, she had so far improved as to be able to get out of bed and walk about the room with the help of sticks.

Oak was continued until in October she was able to walk short distances out of doors. She had very little discomfort and mentally was at peace and very happy.

Unfortunately, the patient was then lost sight of, but when last seen, instead of being an invalid confined to bed and in great pain, she was able to wash and dress herself and walk about in comparative comfort.

CHAPTER XVII

1933-1934. THE LAST YEAR AT CROMER. THE PUBLISH-
ING OF *THE TWELVE HEALERS AND FOUR HELPERS*.
THE PREPARING OF THE REMEDIES OAT, OLIVE AND
VINE

BACH had now found four of the new series of remedies:
Gorse, Oak, Heather and Rock Water; and although
he felt that three more would be necessary to complete
this series, he decided to publish his findings, giving a
detailed description of the uses and preparation of the
first twelve and the newly found four remedies.

He therefore set himself to write the manuscript of
the book *The Twelve Healers and Four Helpers*, which
was published in its present form that autumn of 1933.

He had already worked out the types and states of
mind for which the three other remedies were needed,
and he knew which plants and trees would supply these
needs.

A remedy was required which would help to give
a definite and conscious desire to those in whom ambition,
or the wish to get well and live their lives to the full, was
either lacking, dulled or uncertain; and since he had
become convinced through his great knowledge of
human nature and his own experiences that a definite
purpose in life, a keen interest in some work or whatever
it might be, an alertness and wide-awakeness towards
life in general were vital to the happiness and health of
every individual, this remedy would be of great importance.

So many lacked interest in their daily lives, were
bored, or did uncongenial work, living almost in a state
of coma and performing their duties in a dull, mechanical
way; and this state of mind would at some period of
their lives inevitably affect their physical health, sapping
them of vitality and strength.

The lack of interest and positiveness was apparent not only in the elderly people, but in the young; the many who had ambitions and ideals and knew they were capable of achieving them, but had become side-tracked or were uncertain as to the form their work should take, and had been persuaded by others or influenced by circumstances to live a life devoid of all interest to them.

People of this type, when ill, had no incentive to get well, and made no great efforts towards recovery. Their lack of co-operation and desire to get well was a hindrance indeed to their recovery and, as yet, little had been discovered which would help them.

The plant which contained the necessary medicinal properties to assist such a state of mind, Bach knew to be the wild Oat.

The second remedy was needed for those people who lived their lives to the full, but became so exhausted and weakened by their experiences and sufferings that they lacked the strength to carry on; Bach proved that the flower of the Olive tree contained the life, warmth and strength necessary to re-energise such people and give them back their health.

Finally, the remedy for the definite, capable people who know and achieve their ambitions, have experienced much and, confident themselves in all things, attempt to persuade others to follow their example, was contained in the flower of the grape vine.

In order that the medicinal properties of the Olive and Vine might be extracted from the plants and trees growing in their natural surroundings in the open air, Bach wrote to friends in Switzerland and Italy, asking them to potentise the blooms by the sun method of preparation; and in due course he received the potencies of the Vine from Switzerland and of the Olive and Vine from Italy.

The last remedy, the wild Oat, he found the following

April when he had left Cromer and had gone to the little village of Sotwell in Berkshire. There he found the brome grass (Bromus Asper) growing in the hedge-rows of the village lanes, and he potentised the flowers of the plants one cloudless day in May.

The remainder of the winter of 1933 and the early spring of 1934 Bach spent at Cromer, treating patients and gaining an even greater understanding of the properties of the new remedies.

One combination of three remedies he prepared to use in emergencies, in cases of accident, shock, un-consciousness, great pain, fear or panic; this he called the Rescue Remedy, carrying a bottle of the mixture always in his pocket.

The three remedies in the Rescue Remedy were Rock Rose, Clematis and Impatiens. Rock Rose for emergency, terror, panic and danger; Clematis for unconsciousness, fainting, coma; Impatiens for the state of mental tension and resistance which results in physical contraction and pain.

Later he was to add two more remedies to this number, but as it was, he found the combination of these three remedies invaluable when no other help was available.

On one occasion a man who had been strapped to the mast of a wrecked barge for five hours in a terrible gale was brought ashore by the lifeboat. He was deli-rious, foaming at the mouth, helpless and almost frozen, his life despaired of.

As he was being carried up the sands to a nearby house, Bach repeatedly moistened his lips with the Rescue Remedy, and before the man had been stripped of his clothing and wrapped in warm blankets he was sitting up and in his right mind, asking for a cigarette. He was taken to the hospital, but after a few days' rest he had completely recovered from his dreadful experi-ence.

With the finding of the last three remedies, Bach

knew his researches had ended for the time being; he had perfected the new method of treatment and had now nineteen herbal remedies of great power. He felt that the time had come for him to settle down somewhere in the country not too far from London, build up a practice and let all those who clamoured for his return to town know where they could find and come to him.

Throughout the last four years he had moved about so much and stayed for so short a time in each place that many of his old friends and patients had lost track of him, and letters were frequently lost or only reached him after long delay.

He wished also to get into touch with his former medical colleagues and encourage them to use the new remedies and new method of diagnosis and prescribing. A few staunch friends in the medical profession were already using the remedies and getting excellent results, but the majority, although they looked upon him as a genius for his work as a bacteriologist, found it hard to reconcile themselves to his changed ideas and methods, and to recognise his genius as a herbalist, as he so loved to be called.

Bach hoped to show them that his recent discoveries were of far greater value; that hopeless, incurable cases which would not yield to scientific methods could be cured by the herbal remedies; and that with all his experience of the different branches of medicine, he had found none to equal in results the new method of herbal treatment.

Patients not only regained their physical health, but an added joy and interest in life. Many came to him saying, "I don't know what you have given me, but I feel so well in myself. I have lost all those fears and worries, and life is worth living again."

One patient, who had had to wear a veil for many years owing to a severe face and neck rash, came running to him one day, saying: "You have made me free. I'm just off to buy the most beautiful low-necked evening dress that I can find."

He determined also to continue spreading the knowledge of his discoveries amongst the general public, for more and more people of all classes and professions, not only in England, but in many countries abroad, were using the herbal remedies and obtaining results as good as those of Bach himself.

This latter fact delighted him, and he would often say he envied the lay folk, for they were indeed better prescribers than he. They could concentrate entirely upon the moods and states of mind present in their patients with no conflicting thoughts of the nature of the physical disease to worry them; whereas he, with all those years of medical and scientific experience behind him, found difficulty at times in driving from his mind thoughts of the complications which might arise, or the seriousness of the disease; and the physical symptoms would obtrude in an attempt to blind him to the true guide to the treatment—the patient's mental attitude.

It can, perhaps, be understood by some that for a man who had so extensively explored all scientific and accepted methods of healing, it required at first great courage and implicit trust in his convictions to treat acute and serious conditions with the simple herbs.

No one can quite realise what courage and faith he had when, in the early days of his researches, he tackled such cases; but because of that courage and that faith he proved conclusively the value of his discoveries.

CHAPTER XVIII

CROMER. 1930-1934

THE months spent at Cromer during the past five years had been ones of great happiness and satisfaction for Bach. Most of his research work had been done there, the finding and preparing of eight of the nineteen remedies, and the working out of the principles of the new system of medicine. He had been grateful for the quiet winter months by the sea, for the open-air life and freedom from interruption, noise and crowds, had enabled him to concentrate fully upon the work in hand. For hours he would stroll about the country lanes or along the seashore deep in thought, and he had grown happier and better in health than he had been all his life.

He loved the sea and all pertaining to it, and never tired of watching the fishermen at work or lending them a hand to pull up their boats. Intensely intuitive himself, he admired that quality in the men who lived on and by the sea, for they relied upon their inner knowledge to guide them in their work, knowing so certainly when they should set out with the lines and nets, or drop their pots for crab; some of them going directly to the area, often miles from shore, where they would reap the biggest sea harvest.

Bach's own intuitive powers had become so strongly developed that on occasions he was able to foretell events. Once he warned the fishermen that there would be a gale, and named the day—three weeks ahead—telling them to pull their boats high up the sands upon that day and put their pots and nets in some safe place.

On the day he had named a great storm broke; those who had remembered his warning were saved much worry, but others spent some anxious hours pulling up their boats; and many nets and crab pots were washed away and damaged by the storm.

One night he was awakened by a dream in which he saw a friend of his, a fisherman, in danger. The boat, which was heavy with a big catch of herring, had sprung a leak, and the two men in her were fast asleep. In his dream Bach said to one of them: "Wake up. Wake up," and the man awoke, saw the danger and made for the shore just in time, for the water was flowing in at a great rate.

As Bach awoke, so vivid was the dream and sense of danger that he sprang out of bed and, hurriedly dressing, ran down to the shore, where he saw the boat as pictured in his dream just labouring in. He helped to pull her in, and his friend the fisherman said: "We were asleep, when suddenly I woke up and saw the water running in. We were only just in time. If I had slept much longer we should never have made the shore. How did you come to be here?"

Many such incidents happened in those years. Bach's great compassion and interest in all things and people formed a link between them and him, and by reason of this sympathy he would hear the call for help from any in distress.

Patients would often write to him, or come and tell him afterwards, that during the night when they lay sleepless and in pain he had appeared and placed his hand upon their head or arm and they had immediately gone to sleep.

One cold and stormy night when the lifeboat men stood by ready for a call, and the engineer slept by the lifeboat engine, running her at times to keep her warm, Bach was walking along the seashore when suddenly he heard shouts of distress and fear as though from a great distance, and clearly saw a small ship tossing helplessly in the waves.

He told what he had heard and where he knew the

ship to be, a long way out at sea. The lifeboat crew would have gone in search, but the absence of flares and the usual notifications tied their hands.

Bach was in great distress, and walked the shore all night, for he could still hear the calls for help and see the ship in peril.

The next morning there was washed up on the shore some miles further along the coast the wreckage of a small ship.

The power of healing which Bach possessed had also become more fully developed, and many were conscious that they had but to see him, were it only in the distance, to feel a surge of life and strength flow into them.

Once, during the first year he spent at Cromer, when he was walking in the woods not far from the town, he met a woodsman from whom he asked his way back to the sea. The man was elderly and looked ill, and he began telling Bach the trouble he was having with his mouth, and how his tongue was affected in such a way that he could neither eat nor drink, smoke nor talk in comfort.

The woodsman had no idea the man he spoke to was a doctor, he merely thought he was a summer visitor enjoying a country walk. Bach put his hand on his shoulder, knowing well that the disease from which he suffered had reached an advanced stage, and for which, in the ordinary way, there was little hope of relief, and said to him: "Come and see me some time; I am staying in the town, and we'll have a pint together and drink to your better health."

But it was not until two years later that they met again. Bach was in the street one day when someone stopped him and said: "Sir, I want to tell you that from the day I met you in the wood I have never had one moment's pain or trouble with my tongue," and he opened his mouth and showed his tongue, which was clean and healthy-looking.

One evening he was called to see a child who had a painful wart on one of her fingers, and this had kept her awake and crying for several nights; nothing seemed to ease her. Bach took her on his knee and held the little hand, then said: "Now put her to bed; she'll sleep tonight. Her finger is healed."

Her mother put her to bed, and on looking at the finger found the wart had disappeared.

Often he would feel drawn to go to a certain place at a certain time, and there he would always find his help or advice was needed. Once in the middle of a meal he started up and hurried to the pier-end, and there he found a man so depressed and hopeless that he was about to jump into the sea, and had chosen a time when he thought no one would be about. He had lost his job and could not get another.

Bach told him to have another try and he would be successful, and took him to the local inn for a drink and a good meal. The next morning the man was offered a job and a good salary.

One bitter winter's afternoon Bach was walking through a village some miles from Cromer, when he felt he must get back to the town, and almost running all the way, he arrived to find the lifeboat had returned from rescuing a fisherman who had fallen overboard in the sudden gale which had arisen.

The man was brought ashore unconscious, and the ambulance men were applying artificial respiration. Bach, with his highly developed powers of vision, could see the man's spirit hovering above the body, and he urged the men to continue their efforts. After two hours they felt it was no longer any use attempting to restore breathing and circulation, but Bach asked them to go on, so that, should the spirit decide to return to the body, the process would be made easier.

But in spite of eight hours' unceasing work, during which time the body regained certain vitality and warmth, and the face some colour, the spirit decided not to return to the bodily habitation, and passed up and away.

Only then did Bach consent to the cessation of efforts. None knew what he had seen or that the reason why he had made them continue their work was that so long as the spirit stayed close to the body there was a chance of its deciding to re-enter, thus it was necessary to keep the physical body receptive.

This occurrence—Bach's unceasing care and thought for one of their companions—endeared him to the hearts of all the fishermen, not only of Cromer, but of the neighbouring town from which the drowned man had come, and also served to form a friendlier bond between the men of those two towns.

Bach's implicit trust in his intuition or inner knowledge led to results which others would call miracles or supernatural happenings. He followed the thought that came first into his mind and acted upon it before reason could step in; and again and again, in the small occurrences of his daily life, in the finding and preparing of the herbal remedies, in the healing of disease through his own personal magnetism, and in the saving of life by his foreknowledge of certain events, it was proved to him that through intuition, instinct, man is in touch with the great Source of all Wisdom to Whom nothing is impossible.

CHAPTER XIX

ONE morning in March 1934 Bach left Cromer to wander for the next few weeks through many of the southern counties of England in search of a cottage in some quiet village. He was once more almost at the end of his financial resources, but he felt confident that when he had found the right place in which to settle he would find also some means of earning sufficient money to keep him, for he was determined to hold to his principle of charging no fees to his patients.

How he had lived and been able to do all the things he did during those past four years, travel throughout England and Wales, keep himself clothed, housed and fed, was a miracle indeed. Certain friends had helped him when they could, but the rest he would always say was due to the Protection of the Great Power who watched over him and the work he was given to do.

Most people thought him a wealthy man; that he must have much capital saved from his London practice; and that his whim of charging his patients no fees was merely a rich man's idiosyncrasy. Few knew that often he would have to forgo certain necessities in order to buy the bottles and the brandy with which to make up the doses.

His search led him through Sussex, Kent and Buckinghamshire, but he found nothing suitable until he returned to the Thames valley, which had always held such an attraction for him; there in the village of Sotwell, not far from Wallingford in Berkshire, he took the small house called Mount Vernon.

He moved in in April 1934, and the buying of a few pieces of furniture for the house depleted him of practically all the money he had, but he had no fears for the future, thinking it all but another and exciting adventure.

A few days later, as has been said, he found and prepared the last remedy of the seven helper series—the wild Oat.

He was glad to settle down quietly for the first month or so in his new home, enjoying the peace and beauty of the lovely little village and, above all, revelling in the work of replanning the small garden round the house, for he was becoming increasingly sensitive in mind and body, and his journeyings of the last few weeks had tired him. He let no one know where he was for the time being, neither was it known locally that he was a doctor; thus he was left undisturbed for a few weeks to regain his strength.

During those weeks he wrote the second edition of the book, calling it *The Twelve Healers and Seven Helpers*, and this was published in July 1934.

As he found and proved each new series or group of remedies, Bach lost no time in publishing them, at the same time revising the descriptions of those already in print, and this entailed much work and expense for him. He gained no monetary benefit from the sale of his books *Heal Thyself* and *The Twelve Healers*, for they were sold as inexpensively as possible in order that all might be able to buy them, the small profit from one edition going towards the cost of printing the next.

Neither did he receive any money from the sale of the remedies held by the chemists to whom he had given the mother tinctures, only stipulating that the medicinal preparations should be sold to the public as reasonably as could be. He looked upon these remedies prepared from the flowers of the field as the free gift of the Creator, and as such not to be turned to commercial uses.

The long quiet days spent working in the garden soon restored Bach's strength; his whereabouts then becoming known, patients began to come to him in numbers; and to help him with his work and to deal with his heavy daily correspondence, he trained three lay helpers whom he called his team of workers.

During the earlier part of the summer of 1934 he went to London also once a week to see patients. But he still found the noise and crowds exhausted and depleted him, so he decided to stay at Sotwell and make it the headquarters of the work which he knew, before very many years had passed, would be recognised and the herbal remedies universally used.

It was at this time that one of his team placed the house 'Wellsprings' at his disposal for his work; an old house in the same village of Sotwell, with oak beams across the ceilings and wide, open fireplaces, surrounded by a large garden, an orchard and two fields beyond; and in his leisure moments he set to work to make the furniture for the house, and at the same time to refurnish Mount Vernon.

He made chairs and settles, beds, tables and dressers of elm and deal after his own design, using in most cases wooden pegs in place of nails; then stained them with walnut juice and left them unpolished.

Although he had never done any carpentering before, he made these pieces with rapidity and ease; his love of trees making the handling of wood a great joy to him, and the results were beautiful indeed in their simple dignity.

The work occupied his physical energy and attention, leaving his mind free to think; and this was a great help to him at that period, for the restless feelings which, in the past, had always portended fresh activities and further discoveries, began to take possession of him, and he knew he was on the threshold of new work to be done.

With the finding of the last remedy of the series of nineteen, he had felt that his researches were at an end, but now he realised that other remedies were needed for certain states of mind or moods which had not been included in the first grouping.

As these remedies would not be found until the following spring, he was grateful for the carpentering work which absorbed his energy throughout the winter months.

He was to gain his knowledge of the second nineteen remedies and their uses in an entirely different way from that in which he discovered the first group of remedies.

For some days before the discovery of each one he suffered himself from the state of mind for which that particular remedy was required, and suffered it to such an intensified degree that those with him marvelled that it was possible for a human being to suffer so and retain his sanity; and not only did he pass through terrible mental agonies, but certain states of mind were accompanied by a physical malady in its most severe form.

Such experiences needed courage and faith beyond the average, for although Bach knew that with the discovery of the right remedy that particular mental and bodily torture would cease, yet there were nineteen to find, and with each great suffering to bear.

His tremendous courage and his desire to find the means of relieving the sufferings of others alone sustained him; and although at times he could not stand or even sit in comfort, he never rested nor spared himself. He continued to see his patients, deal with his correspondence, and search the countryside for the new remedies, sometimes on foot or by bicycle, and at other times when he was too ill to use his legs, by car.

In March 1935 he found the first remedy of the new series, the Cherry Plum.

For some days before he had been suffering from severe inflammation of the frontal sinuses, an agonising pain across the cheekbones, and a blinding and persistent headache; the pain was so intense that he felt desperate, as though life was no longer possible without loss of reason.

He knew he must be on the verge of discovering the remedy for this state of mind, and early one morning he went out to wander about the fields and lanes looking for it. Then it was he came upon a hedge white with the blossoms of the Cherry Plum, and he picked some of the flowering sprigs and took them back with him.

The plant is of a tough and woody nature, and the sun in early spring has not the strength it gains later in the year, so he decided to boil the flowering sprigs in water on the fire.

This he did, letting them simmer for an hour; when it had cooled he strained off the fluid and took a few drops of the remedy. Almost at once his mental agony ceased, and with it the physical pain; by the next morning he was perfectly well.

During the following six months he found the remaining eighteen remedies, choosing the flowers and young leaf sprays of eleven trees: the common elm, the pine, larch, willow, aspen; hornbeam, sweet chestnut, beech; crab apple and walnut; the young swelling bud and the red and white flowers of the horse chestnut trees; of three bushes: holly, honeysuckle and wild rose; and of two plants: Star of Bethlehem and the wild Mustard.

The White Chestnut alone he potentised by the sun method, the others were prepared by boiling; the water strained off when cold and put into bottles with an equal amount of brandy to preserve them.

The last remedy of this new series he potentised in August of the same year, and then he published a short account of his findings in leaflet form which was inserted into the book *The Twelve Healers and Seven Helpers*.

The strain of the last six months had been very great indeed; remedy after remedy had been found and prepared in quick succession, and the mental and physical agony he had experienced before the discovery of each had been so severe that he was left very exhausted and weak.

Although the discovery of these remedies appears so simple, yet only those working and living with him could tell of the almost superhuman courage and determination which he needed and which he possessed to enable him to endure these experiences.

For many days, and this during the hottest part of the summer, his body was completely covered by a virulent rash which burned and irritated incessantly; and for some weeks his legs were ulcerated, raw from knee to ankle; his hair came out and his sight almost failed. Before the finding of another remedy his face was swollen and extremely painful. A severe hæmorrhage exhausted him and the bleeding did not cease until the remedy for the mental state he was passing through was found.

Not only did he pass through the states of mind for which the new remedies were needed and suffer physically so greatly, but, such was his sensitive condition, he was aware of the disease or complaint of the next patient who was to visit him sometimes hours before that patient reached the house.

He would contract the symptoms of the disease himself for some few hours previously, and this, although so distressing for him, gave him such an understanding and sympathy with his patients that they immediately gained certainty of help, reassured by his intimate knowledge of their condition.

Yet in spite of the great mental and physical suffering he experienced during those months, he never lost his intense interest in the affairs of the village, nor ceased his efforts in bringing the joy and happiness to his fellow-men he knew to be so essential to their health and well-being.

He would arrange sing-songs at the village inn,

singing his favourite songs to fill up some gap in the programme, laughing and joking with all his friends and making sure the evening began with a free round of drinks at his expense. His interest in the cricket and football clubs took a practical form as well, and during the football matches in the field he lent to the club he was always to be seen with a smile and cheery word for everyone. An outstanding figure, striding along with his spaniel Lulu, staff in hand, bare-headed and bearded —for he had grown a beard during the last few months— radiating happiness and companionship.

I sprang up from my body
   For all the world to see,
But they looked down with tear-filled eyes
   At that which wasn't me.

I shot up to the Heavens,
   And then swooped down again,
I shouted out in sheer delight
   With all my might and main.

I wrapped my arms around them,
   Those ones who mourned so,
I said, "Oh, know my happiness,
   Do try, do try to know!"

Then one looked up from mourning
   O'er that which was not I,
And said in breathless wonder,
   "I feel that he is nigh,
I heard a little whisper,
   I know it was his voice,
He said, 'Oh, know my happiness,
   Rejoice with me, rejoice!' "

                            Mary Tabor.

CHAPTER XX

SOTWELL. THE BOOK *THE TWELVE HEALERS AND OTHER REMEDIES*. THE LECTURE 'THE HEALING HERBS.' LAST ILLNESS AND DEATH OF EDWARD BACH

ALTHOUGH Bach was still very tired and weakened from his experiences of the last six months, he had not much opportunity for rest. Patients increased in numbers, keeping him and his team of workers fully occupied; many came to be instructed in the use of the herbal remedies, and letters arrived from all parts of the world from people who were getting excellent results.

This gave him much satisfaction, for the great aim of all his work had been to find remedies and a method of treatment which could be used by everyone, were they possessed of medical knowledge or not. He felt very strongly that the healing of the sick should not be in the hands of a limited number of persons, but that it was the right of all who had the wish to be of help in cases of illness.

Therefore, when he received a notification form with a marked paragraph referring to unqualified assistants from the General Medical Council in January 1936, he determined to remind the Council of his views upon the matter. If they decided to strike his name off the Medical Register it would make no difference to him; indeed, he rather welcomed the idea, for he wished to be known as a herbalist, and always called himself one; and he would still continue to teach the people how they could heal themselves.

He wrote and sent the following letter on January 8th, 1936:

To the President of the General Medical Council.
DEAR SIR,

Having received the notification of the Council concerning working with unqualified assistants, it is only honourable to inform you that I am working with several, and shall continue to do so.

As I have previously informed the Council, I consider it the duty and privilege of any physician to teach the sick and others how to heal themselves.

I leave it entirely to your discretion as to the course you take.

Having proved that the herbs of the field are so simple to use and so wonderfully effective in their healing powers, I deserted orthodox medicine.

Yours sincerely,

EDWARD BACH.

He was fully prepared to hear by return that his name was to be removed from the Medical Register; it would mean that he and his assistants could no longer visit patients in their homes, but this was of no great importance, for he had found the patients who gained the greatest benefit were those who made the effort to come to him.

He also sent the same day a copy of this letter with a covering note to each of his lay workers in other parts of the country:

"Enclosed a copy of a letter sent to-day to the General Medical Council, which will shortly prohibit any of our team from visiting houses.

"The sick will have to come to us, or parents or relatives report to us the nature of the case. This we know is very right, as it is those who make an effort who get well. They are the kind of people who took up a flooring because the throng was so great that it was the only way to reach a Healer."

Having sent these letters he forgot all about the

matter in the work which was increasing so rapidly. Weeks and months passed, but no reply came from the General Medical Council, neither did he receive any further communication from them.

During the summer of 1936 he began to write the manuscript of the third edition of his book, which he named *The Twelve Healers and Other Remedies*, and this was published in September of that year.

He took infinite pains to revise the descriptions of the first nineteen remedies and to add the simplest possible account of the others, until he was satisfied that all could understand their meaning and recognise the types he had depicted.

When the manuscript had been sent to the publishers, he set to work to write a paper on the method of treatment and prescribing of the herbs, calling it 'The Healing Herbs', for he felt that the best way to spread the knowledge of the remedies amongst the general public was by means of a lecture tour. He planned that he and his team of workers should go from place to place giving the address, and he gave the first lecture himself in the nearby town of Wallingford, on the day of his fiftieth birthday, September 24th, 1936.

Towards the end of October his strength began seriously to fail; his body, which had been so true a friend to him, could no longer stand the strain of further action, and he was forced to stay in bed.

But he did not cease to work; under his supervision his three assistants dealt with his large correspondence, gave his lecture in towns and villages, and prescribed for the patients.

He trained his team with great care, for now that his work of finding the herbs and perfecting the new method of the treatment of disease was completed, he wished to leave its application in their hands and in the hands of all those who, scattered throughout the world, were already using his system of herbal medicine.

His whole time and attention could then be given to his future work, for he knew he had more to find out in connection with the healing of disease. He had no knowledge as yet what that work might be, or whether it would be done on earth or on another plane.

Life, to him, was continuous: an unbroken stream, uninterrupted by what we call death, which merely heralded a change of conditions; and he was convinced that some work could only be done under earthly conditions, whilst spiritual conditions were necessary for certain other work.

His marvellous vitality, his ability to make light of all his sufferings and his unbounded sense of fun and interest in all things led those around him to hope he would soon recover, but he gradually became weaker. At one time he rallied and began to regain his appetite and strength, but this brief rally did not last, and in the evening of November 27th, 1936, he died in his sleep.

The years of his life had been short, but during those fifty years he had worked without ceasing and with but one aim in view: to find a pure and simple way of healing the sick. Then, having accomplished all that was possible for him to do on earth, he gladly laid down his physical body to continue his work in another sphere, content that those who had been with him would be unceasing in their efforts to spread the knowledge of the healing herbs.

His whole life had been one of service and of giving. His generosity was such that he left few personal belongings; of clothes he had barely more than those he wore, for he had given them all away; of money he had just over £50, part of a £100 legacy recently left him, and this he had planned to use in extending the scope of the work.

It had always been his custom to destroy any notes made during the course of his researches directly he had reached the final conclusion and published the result.

He felt in this way there would be no conflicting accounts to puzzle the learner; his aim being to make the healing of disease a simple matter, and so remove the fear present in the minds of most at the thought of illness.

He would say: "I want to make it as simple as this: 'I am hungry, I will go and pull a lettuce from the garden for my tea; I am frightened and ill, I will take a dose of Mimulus.' "

CHAPTER XXI

RESULTS OBTAINED BY THE THIRTY-EIGHT HERBAL REMEDIES

FROM 1930 until 1936 Bach used the herbal remedies alone in the treatment of all cases of disease and sickness that came to him, and the results fully justified his conviction that the true healing agents are contained in the beneficent plants and trees of Nature; a fact which had been recognised centuries ago, when herbs were the only means of healing used by mankind.

Moreover, his ambition to find pure and simple remedies which would assist in the process of healing with no painful or distressing reactions in the patient had been accomplished; for the thirty-eight herbs heal gently and surely, and as there are no poisonous plants amongst them there is no fear of ill effects from overdoses or incorrect prescriptions.

These remedies can also, if desired, be used in conjunction with other treatments and medicines, for this does not detract from their beneficial effects; and the method of prescribing is so simple that they can be kept in the home and used by everyone, as were, and still are in certain parts, the remedies of Culpepper and other old herbalists.

With the help of the additional nineteen remedies Bach obtained excellent results in cases which had not fully responded to the remedies in the first group, and he was satisfied that, throughout his years of research and experience in orthodox medicine, he had found nothing to be compared with the curative powers of these thirty-eight herbs.

Long-standing and obstinate complaints yielded to treatment, sometimes in a remarkably short space of time; and patients whose lives had been made a burden through such minor complaints as continual colds, headaches, chilblains, or suffered greatly from over-strain, worry, fears and depressions, although not physically ill, regained not only good health, but a feeling of well-being and happiness they had never expected to attain.

One man, suffering from the after-effects of shell-shock, could not bear to be in a closed room, jumped at the slightest noise, and was left shaken and speechless when cars passed him in the street. Every night he had terrifying dreams from which he woke up shouting, trembling and bathed in perspiration, and this made him dread the approach of bedtime. He was extremely restless, in continual dread of something he could not define, and feared he might do something desperate if his condition did not improve.

His physical health was poor; he suffered from severe indigestion, flatulence and constipation, with a persistent backache.

He was given a prescription of the following remedies: Rock Rose for his terror; Cherry Plum for his fear of doing something desperate; Aspen for his fear of the unknown; Mimulus for his fear of people and noises; Sweet Chestnut for the almost unbearable mental anguish; Scleranthus for his unbalanced, uncertain state of mind; and Agrimony for his restlessness.

The following week he reported that he felt calmer; he had passed three nights without dreaming and the pain in the back was less severe. The prescription was repeated, and the patient was not seen for one month, when he reported great improvement.

He had had only one terrifying dream during that period, his indigestion was definitely better, the bowels working normally, and—most important of all to him —he found he could now eat his dinner in the canteen of his place of work instead of having to go away and be by himself. He felt much more confident of cure, but traffic and sudden noises still worried him.

The remedies Mimulus, Agrimony, Aspen, Honey-suckle and Larch were then prescribed. Honeysuckle was added because he was inclined to let his thoughts dwell too much on the past and the origin of his condition, and Larch to help him regain complete confidence in himself.

The patient was not then seen for eight months, when he reported he had been feeling so well that he had not felt the need of more doses. He had entirely lost his fears and terrors, was sleeping well, and felt happier and more contented than he had done for twenty years. He considered himself cured except for occasional bouts of depression and a slight return of the indigestion.

The remedies Scleranthus, Mimulus, Rock Water, Gentian and Mustard were then given: Scleranthus to maintain his regained poise and certainty; Mimulus for his fear of eating certain foods in case they should cause him discomfort; Rock Water because he had developed into a man with rigid principles, very strict in his way of life; and Gentian and Mustard for his bouts of depression and gloom.

This combination of remedies was repeated for three weeks, and he continued coming at intervals during the next few months, for, although he felt so well, he said it gave him confidence to know he had a bottle of his remedies in the house.

Another man had been gassed during the Great War, and his breathing was still difficult at times; he also had severe attacks of gastric pain and sickness, which greatly interfered with his work.

He was a man of very decided views, extremely capable, but slightly domineering in his manner; these characteristics indicated the remedy Vine. He resented his disability, blaming the circumstances of its origin, for which he was given Willow; and past events formed the greater part of his conversation, indicating the remedy Honeysuckle.

During the attacks he became frightened—Mimulus; undecided—Schleranthus; suffered from intense depression—Mustard.

These six remedies were taken for four weeks, and by the end of that time his condition had improved so greatly that he was filled with hope, and had lost his fears and depression. He continued the treatment throughout the winter months, which were trying ones for his condition, but through which he passed, to his surprise, with very little discomfort.

The prescriptions were varied according to his changing states of mind; at one time he became very worried, fearing his wife was seriously ill, and this caused a return of the gastric pain and difficulty in breathing. The excessive over-concern for another indicated the remedy Red Chestnut, which he was given together with Clematis, for he had lost all interest in his work, going about in a dreamy state, his thoughts continually with his wife.

Another time, after an intensive spell of work, he felt so weak and exhausted that he had no strength left to carry on, and his mind became so tired that he could not stop thinking about his work, continually carrying on mental conversations and puzzling over problems. For the first state he was given Olive, and for the latter White Chestnut, and with the help of these two remedies he soon regained his strength and normal peace of mind.

By the end of the year he had entirely forgotten his original complaints, coming for treatment occasionally for colds, slight rheumatic pains in the legs and the like.

A lady had suffered from varicose ulcers on both ankles for many years; they healed at times, but almost immediately broke out again. The legs and feet were swollen, very discoloured, and she complained of continual and very distressing irritation. She was hopeless of cure, resigned to her condition, but she thought she would try the herbal remedies.

Gorse for the hopelessness, Wild Rose for her resigned state of mind, and Agrimony for the torture of the irritation were given for several weeks. The patient became more hopeful and the irritation was less severe, although there was no change in the swelling or sign of the ulcers closing up.

She felt very unhappy about her legs, considering them unclean, and for this state of mind Crab Apple was added to the prescription, also the remedy Chicory, for she was of the type who worried unnecessarily over her children and household affairs.

Within a few weeks the ulcer on the right ankle healed over, but there was still much swelling and discoloration and no improvement in the left ankle.

The patient seemed to have lost all ambition and real interest in life, her disability had limited her and prevented her from doing all the things she wanted to do, and there seemed no active desire to get well. This clearly indicated the remedy Oat, which she was given alone.

The results were almost immediate and improvement astonishing. She reported that the ulcer on the left ankle was getting smaller, discharging less, the swelling and discoloration was subsiding on both legs and the irritation had ceased.

Oat was continued for several weeks with increasing improvement until both ulcers had healed, and but a slight swelling around the ankles remained. The improvement was maintained.

A gardener had suffered from dermatitis on both hands for some weeks; the skin was cracked and rough, with large raw places on the backs of the hands, and an almost unbearable irritation. He had tried many treatments with no lasting benefit.

The man was happy, cheerful, energetic, always laughing and singing at his work, hiding his worries from his wife and friends, which clearly indicated the remedy Agrimony. He was also given White Chestnut, for the thought of loss of work was ever present in his mind and he could not shake it off; Holly and Impatiens as he felt impatient and irritable with others, although he did his best to hide it; and Elm, for he was keenly conscious of his responsibilities and at times wondered whether he would be able to fulfil them.

These five remedies were given as a medicine and lotion, and the patient was not seen again for some weeks, when he came to report that his hands had completely healed. Within a few days of taking the medicine he had been able to discard the bandages which he had been forced to wear, the irritation both physical and mental had ceased, and the skin of his hands was soft and pliable and healthy with no sign of the complaint. He has had no recurrence.

A labourer had suffered from dermatitis on both hands for several years; when seen, the hands were in a terrible state, raw and painful, the nails almost destroyed and suppurating, the irritation intense; he also had patches of the same complaint on his legs.

He was utterly tired out through lack of sleep, which made him intolerant and vexed with his condition and with other people; he had tried many treatments to cleanse himself of his trouble, and his failure to do so depressed and discouraged him.

Therefore the following remedies were prescribed and given as medicine and lotion: Olive for the exhaustion; Beech and Holly for the mental irritation and intolerance; Crab Apple to cleanse and Gentian for the depression and discouragement.

He came at intervals for three months, improvement occurring rapidly in the legs and general health, more gradually in the hands. The prescription was varied according to his changes of mood. At one period he was filled with self-pity and suffered from fits of intense depression and gloom, for which he was given Chicory and Mustard. After a slight relapse he began to feel hopeless and lost his interest in his work, when Gorse and Clematis helped him and again set him on the road to recovery.

At the end of three months his hands were cured, and he said he felt better in health and spirits than he had done for several years.

A boy of ten years had had periodic attacks of urti-caria on the back, neck and chest for two years. He was a cheerful lad who made light of his trouble, although the discomfort and irritation during an attack kept him awake at night and impaired his general health. His temperament indicated the remedy Agrimony, which was given as a medicine and lotion, and within a few days the condition had cleared up. He had a slight return in two months' time which was quickly cured with the same remedy, and since then—a period of five years—he has had no recurrence.

A middle-aged man, crippled with rheumatoid arthritis of both hips, knees, ankles and wrists, had given up hope of recovery; he managed to get about with the help of two sticks, but was in continual pain. His joints were badly deformed, his muscles atrophied and his general health poor. He suffered from constipation and piles which irritated incessantly and bled frequently.

Although he had great difficulty in getting about, he continued his work, which necessitated being on his feet many hours a day, and he tried every treatment possible in the hope of finding some slight relief, but with very little success.

He was of a nervous disposition, over-concerned lest his family and work should suffer through him; blaming himself for his illness, and working too hard, which further weakened him and caused him to become irritable and touchy.

The following remedies were given: Gorse for his hopelessness of cure; Red Chestnut for his over-concern for others; Pine for self-blame; Vervian for his intensity and over-strain; Centaury for the weakness; Mimulus for his nervousness; and Impatiens for his impatience and irritability.

These remedies he took for a month and was delighted with the result. He had less pain, could walk further with greater freedom in the hip and knee joints.

He began to hope that he might get well, but in spite of his improvement he had times of doubt and depression, for which he was given Gentian and Mustard; and of lack of confidence, which indicated the remedy Larch.

His work necessitated his travelling about the country, so that sometimes there were long intervals between his visits to Sotwell, but progress was maintained, and he finally discarded his sticks, walking in reasonable comfort for three miles. He could stand almost upright, having regained full extension in the hips. The left knee was still painful and stiff, but the wrists were practically normal and he had put on weight, although the leg muscles were still wasted and weak.

He then became impatient to get well quickly— indicating the remedy Impatiens—and continually tried other treatments, ointments and patent medicines in addition to the herbal remedies, spending a good deal of time and money over them; his former experiences not having proved to him their ineffectiveness, and for this phase he was given the remedy Chestnut Bud.

Within a year of the first dose he felt a different man. He could walk five miles without sticks on London pavements; the constipation had cleared up and the piles rarely troubled him; he was sleeping and eating well, happier than he had been for years. The left knee was still slightly painful and stiff and the muscles of his legs had not yet regained their normal strength, otherwise he was doing a full day's work without undue fatigue.

A young girl suffered from continual colds which

she found difficult to shake off and which affected her general health, making her feel her work was too much for her strength, although she pluckily carried on.

Two or three remedies were given without much result; then Hornbeam was tried, and after one bottle of this remedy her health improved in a really remarkable way, and she passed the rest of that winter and the following one without any sign of a cold.

An elderly man had had a sudden and sharp attack of sciatica five weeks before. The pain was very severe and he could neither walk, sit nor lie in comfort. The shock of the sudden attack had made him nervous and the continual pain caused him to be very irritable. He had undergone treatment which had relieved the acute symptoms, but he still had pain down the back of the thigh and calf, worse at night and when sitting down.

He was given Star of Bethlehem for the shock of the sudden attack, Larch and Mimulus to give him back his confidence and remove his fear of using the leg in case the acute symptoms returned; and Impatiens and Vervain for his state of irritability and over-tension.

Within a week the pain in the thigh had gone; he had good nights, but still complained of pain in the calf and a lack of strength in the leg muscles. He was restless and still impatient with the pain.

Impatiens, Vervain, Mimulus and Larch were continued; Agrimony for the restlessness and Hornbeam to give him strength were added to the prescription, and after three weeks' treatment he was quite free of pain, was sleeping and walking normally, and driving a car for long distances in comfort.

This girl of eighteen had suffered from epileptic fits since birth, sometimes two or three attacks a week, at other times a month would pass without any trouble.

She was physically well and strong and wanted very much to go out to work, but her mother thought it would be bad for her and kept her at home doing nothing. The girl had a sense of frustration, lost interest and lacked confidence in herself, which did not help her condition.

The remedies Clematis, Scleranthus, Larch and Walnut were given and she took them for seven weeks, during which time she had three attacks, each one in the early morning whilst still in bed.

Clematis was given for the state of unconsciousness during the attack and for her loss of interest in life; Scleranthus for her uncertainty and lack of mental balance; Larch to give her back her confidence; and Walnut because she had allowed her own ambitions to be frustrated.

She continued under treatment for ten months, during which time the prescriptions were varied according to the moods present. Centaury was added at one time to give her back the strength to overcome her difficulty and to help her to stand alone, and for some few weeks she was given Oat as a single remedy in order to increase her desire to make some use of her life.

Five months passed without an attack, then she had a slight one, again in the early morning, which caused her to feel discouraged; Gentian and Honeysuckle were added to the medicine, the latter remedy to help her to forget the past, and she soon regained her hopefulness and confidence.

Her character gradually became more positive, and she finally decided to look out for some work, feeling confident she would be able to do it. She took a post in the neithbouring town as nursery maid to three children, and continued coming for doses during the following month, merely as a precautionary measure.

When last seen she had had no more attacks, and had changed from a weak, shy, rather hysterical girl into a calm, confident and happy young woman.

CHAPTER XXII

EDWARD BACH: PERSONAL IMPRESSIONS

"My acquaintance with Edward Bach began in the early twenties of this century while he was acting as Pathologist to the London Homœopathic Hospital. We quickly became friends, for I was at once interested in the quickness and originality of his mind, and very willingly began to work along his lines of thought.

"I was able to help in relating his bacteriological work to current homœopathic practice and conceptions of disease, and can never sufficiently express my gratitude to Bach for all that I learnt from him.

"Later we had rooms at the same house and saw a great deal of one another, and our association resulted in the writing of the book *Chronic Disease*. That led to his friendship with Dr. Dishington and Dr. Paterson of Glasgow, and they again added to the scope of the work and expanded its fundamental conceptions at an International Congress in 1927; three of us presented a joint thesis on these matters.

"Some little time after this Bach began to develop the ideas with which his memory is now most closely associated. He came to think that much of his earlier teaching was defective and abandoned bacteriology.

"I have not been able to follow his thought easily in these later years, and he thought me, I fear, slow and reactionary.

"But I want to leave on record my affection and respect for one who had something of the quality that is called genius, and was throughout a staunch and generous comrade and friend. I have seldom known one more free from any taint of self-seeking, more single-minded in altruism, more courageous in asserting what he felt to be the truth.

"The world is much the poorer for the loss of Edward Bach."

C. E. WHEELER, M.D., B.S., B.Sc.

In Edward Bach genius was combined with a joyousness and simplicity of nature, a great humility and lack of self-pride in his achievements which endeared him to all those with whom he worked or came in contact.

His striking personality, his intuitive knowledge and understanding of human nature, his certainty of his own purpose in life and disregard of all that might interfere with that mission, made him one of those outstanding characters who are remembered and loved for themselves and their work throughout the world's history.

Of average height—although he had the appearance of being much taller— broad-shouldered, with fair hair and fine brown eyes, his intense vitality and alertness attracted attention wherever he might be.

The kindliness and extreme generosity of his nature were shown both by the way in which he explained and published every detail of his discoveries so that all might benefit from them, and by his ever-readiness to help those in distress with medical advice, with money, or with the actual work of his own hands.

Mr. Jack Davies, one of his friends amongst the fishermen of Norfolk, said of him: "I liked him so much for the way he was always ready at any time, whether night or day, to give a helping hand to anyone, in any shape or form. Rich or poor, it did not matter to him."

His generosity and entire lack of acquisitiveness caused him to be a poor man from the material point of view throughout his life, but in some miraculous manner his pockets were never empty when necessity arose. He would often laugh over the fact that the first holes and rents to appear in his clothes were in the pockets, so well were they used.

New clothes were anathema to him; he would go

about in any old garment so long as it was comfortable, and when he required a new suit it would be of the thinnest material possible and made to fit him very loosely. He could as little bear to have the freedom of his bodily actions restricted by tight clothing as he could stand interference with the purpose of his life.

Though he occasionally wore a hat in London it was a continual irritation to him, and it never stayed on his head for long. Those who knew him then remember the small unconscious shakes and jerks with which he strove to free himself of the slight weight; and when he left London he also left the hat behind, and never wore one again until he bought himself a sou'wester for the stormy weather by the sea.

Never for one moment did he consider his personal appearance, and when remonstrated with, as happened to him at times, he would say if people wished to meet *him* they must take him as he was, but if they wished to meet a suit of clothes, he would send them one with pleasure.

Once he was noticed walking along a country lane with a new football under his arm, as usual in his old and well-worn clothes. A passer-by, not knowing who he was, went to a shop in the nearby town to enquire whether they had lost a football.

On being asked the reason, he said: "I saw a tramp walking along with a new one under his arm," and described his appearance.

"Why, that is Dr. Bach," the shopkeeper hastened to explain. "He has just bought the ball to give to the village lads. He is always doing things like that."

The passer-by recounted this tale himself when later he came as a patient and derived great benefit from Bach's herbal remedies.

Everywhere Bach wandered during the last seven years of his life, both in towns and villages, people of every class welcomed him, confided in him and made a friend of him. His great understanding of men and women, his broad-minded individuality appealed to all types.

Mr. B. A. Barnett, his laboratory assistant at the London Homœopathic Hospital and at the laboratory in Park Crescent, describes him thus:

"Dr. Bach was the kindest man I ever met. He was so good to all, rich or poor, and he always had a smile for everyone.

"As regards the research work, the Doctor was always at it, and I have often wakened him up at 8.30 a.m. at Park Crescent to see a patient, because he had been up all night waiting to take a culture out of the incubator. That goes to show how he loved his patients, and his great ambition was to see everyone in the very best of health.

"Whatever I wanted as regards apparatus he never said no."

Edward Bach kept his own individuality wherever he might be, playing darts in the village inn, talking to the fisherfolk on the seashore, lecturing to some medical society, or helping and advising patients in every station of life.

His genius was entirely natural and unassuming, and his great sense of humour and fun gave him a tremendous capacity for enjoyment, both of work and play.

During his busy years in London he had kept himself fit with boxing and rowing on the lake in Regent's Park in the very early mornings, and on wintry days he was a familiar figure flinging handfuls of sprats to the hungry seagulls and bread to his other little friends, the ducks and sparrows in the park.

He possessed the great gift of making all who came to him feel they were his equal and more than equal; and, above all, he was one of those rare individuals who awaken in others a renewed sense of joy and interest in life, and a quickening of their observation and appreciation of the beauty in all around.

To him life was a glorious and joyous adventure, and one in which to gain all the experience and knowledge possible.

Ever direct in speech, fearless of giving offence when he wished to emphasise the truth, he always refused to argue or reason with others. Quick to decide and act upon decision, never discouraged nor swayed by other people's opinions, his single-minded purposefulness gained from some misunderstanding, but from the great majority a deep and fasting affection.

He had the ability to perceive and instantly act upon the truth of any new knowledge he gained through his researches and, as these were sometimes revolutionary and unorthodox according to ordinary standards, they often aroused scepticism and doubt at first in those who were not so ready to learn or so quick in perception.

His intense desire to help others to understand and learn as quickly as he did himself sometimes made him impatient at slowness, but this mood would not last long, for he was possessed of infinite patience; and although he was quick to anger at injustice, unhesitatingly voicing it and siding with the weaker, he would encourage the weak one to fight his own battles and so regain his self-esteem.

For such a man as Bach, one who stood apart from his fellows by reason of his genius, life was not easy.

His intuitive faculties and highly developed sensitiveness of mind and body caused him at times to suffer intensely, and he experienced pain and disease, difficulties and hardships to the uttermost limit; but these he passed through with courage and gratitude, for he felt that through his own experiences he would eventually make the way easier for others. It was said of him that he slew seven dragons so that others might be encouraged to slay one.

In one of his notebooks he wrote: "No man should be a leader amongst others for any length of time unless

he were more expert in his special branch of knowledge
than his followers, whether it be army, statesmanship or
whatever. It therefore follows to be a leader against
trouble, difficulties, disease, persecution and so forth,
the leader must still have a greater knowledge, a more
intimate experience, than, pray God, his followers
need ever suffer."

Bach had need of his own courage and faith, for the
last seven years of his life were lonely ones for him; his
work, during that period, was based entirely on the
knowledge that he gained intuitively, and for such the
world has little understanding or encouragement,
needing causes, scientific provings, before it is ready to
believe. But the practical results of his researches, the
relief of so many sufferers, was sufficient reward for him.

"I first met Edward Bach at the International Homœopathic Congress in 1929. This meeting was the beginning of a friendship lasting until the day of his death.
During these years I had the privilege of keeping in
touch with him either personally or by letter, and in
this way sharing with him each new discovery.

"One characteristic of his work was his unselfish
desire to help humanity; he wanted nothing for himself.
The finding of each new remedy filled him with joy and
thankfulness to the Giver of all. He considered himself
only as the instrument through which the remedies
came. In one letter, after discussing the healing properties of a new remedy, he wrote: 'This is not my work.
All praise be to Him who gives us knowledge for the
relief of mankind.'

"Bach has gone from our vision, but his work lives
on, and only those who worked with him know the
great value of his discoveries."

F. J. WHEELER, M.R.C.S., L.R.C.P.

The keynote of Edward Bach's life was simplicity

and it was also the keynote of his final work—the new system of herbal medicine.

His personal tastes were all simple. He joyed in little things, and nothing that needed care and attention was too unimportant for his notice. He loved the country villages, the sing-songs at the inns, working in his garden, helping the fishermen haul up their boats, exploring the countryside and the river banks for new plants or flowers.

There were many aspects of his character; tremendous gentleness and compassion, great strength and purpose-fulness, an idealism which was yet intensely practical, quick to anger, but the anger as quickly over; and as was once written of him, a man "above all to inspire one with confidence when things go crooked."

But the true description of him is contained in a single word—naturalness.

On all occasions, and no matter where or with whom he happened to be, he was absolutely and entirely himself. He wasted no thought on the opinions of others, for he kept one great Example ever before his eyes—that of his Master, Christ, who combined in Himself all qualities, manliness and gentleness and strength to face the truth.

Bach lived his life without pretence or sham, true to his own nature, and by his example encouraged all who knew him to recognise the greatness and beauty that lay within themselves.

"Those of us who had the privilege of being closely associated with Dr. Edward Bach during the latter years of his life can never be sufficiently grateful for the experience.

"In this healing work which he gave to us, and which we continue in his name, we gratefully acknowledge his inspiration and help.

"The keynote is HAPPINESS. He knew so well that

happiness uplifts and opens the way to good health, just as unhappiness, in all its forms, paves the way for disease.

"The great destroyers of happiness are the states of mind, such as fear, anxiety, depression, impatience, irritability, grief and so on.

"But he was not content just to point out these things. He knew the futility of attempting to remove the fears of a terror-stricken patient by words alone, or how useless it is to tell a patient enveloped in gloom to be happy. Most of us know how difficult it is to shake off these adverse moods.

"Dr. Bach was above all things practical, so that great was his joy when he discovered that there were certain herbs and trees of Nature endowed with the power to remove our fears, our anxieties, our impatience and such-like, and to assist in bringing back to us the joy of living.

"And with the return of happiness comes the return to good health, for this alteration in the state of mind of a patient always precedes an alteration in his physical body, and the disease, no matter what it may be, just drops away.

"Nearly always a patient remarks after having been given the herbs: 'I feel so much better in myself,' and we know then that soon the patient will be physically better.

"This system of herbal healing given us by Dr. Bach is a return to the real healing, because not only is the physical state relieved, but what is of far greater importance, the mind is healed and the whole being uplifted and made happy."

ROBERT VICTOR BULLEN.

DR. EDWARD BACH: AN APPRECIATION

Dr. Edward Bach created one of the most important, beautiful and comprehensive systems of holistic therapy and healing. It is unique in many ways, perhaps firstly and most importantly because he recognized what has become increasingly rare in twentieth century medical practice, that is the spirtual and mental etiology of all suffering and disease. He searched for natural ways of relieving mental and physical disharmony so that the healing life energy within the body, the *vis medicatrix naturae* of Hippocrates, the Archaeus of Paracelsus, could be enhanced and mobilized to enable the healing process to begin — the true healing process, that which starts from within.

In this Bach was guided by his homoeopathic studies. Hahnemann had taught that healing commenced with the activation and enhancement of what he referred to as the vital force, and like Hahnemann, Bach searched for small doses of natural substances which would activate this vital force. He was guided to natural living plants rather than, as Hahnemann had been, to a wide variety of substances of the animal, vegetable and mineral kingdoms.

Bach was looking for healing from nature. He believed with Paracelsus that, "All nature is like one single apothecary's shop, covered only with the roof of heaven; and only One Being works the pestle as far as the world extends." The system that Dr. Bach developed from this seems to me, of all of medicine, the most loving and the most poetic.

From his deep love of nature and loving observations of man he recognized the relationship between certain plants and people's personalities and from this his system developed.

He turned away from Hahnemann's somewhat mechanical methods which destroy the God-given plant in the process of making the remedy. He first collected the vital energy of the plant from its dew, as Paracelsus had done centuries earlier. Then he collected it through spring water and sunshine. Thus he developed his healing system in a most complete and beautiful relationship with the healing powers around us in nature.

He then treated the precise spiritual and psychological disharmonies with the specific remedies he had now prepared so as to re-balance and enhance the life energy. Spiritual and mental and physical sickness were thus relieved. Perhaps even more importantly if the disharmonies were corrected at an early stage physical disease would be prevented and the way would now be opened to positive health.

Bach's life work itself became a testament, the path of true medicine and healing for us all. It was a path not of medical fame or prestige or fortune but of doing his work as best he could, obeying his calling, forsaking the worldly for his aim, developing his goal. He was thus free to research and treat as he felt led and as a result this beautiful system has been handed on to us.

The true medical advance will always be simple, natural, beautiful, loving and poetic. This was very difficult in Bach's day and today it has become exceedingly rare as we are now faced with increasing regulation and the drive to conformity. The time of true far-reaching medical pioneering, such as Bach did, may well be over.

His is of course not the only way to holistic treatment, but it is a true and definite way. Used wisely and with respect the remedies can be of inestimable value. Their power for good is invaluable, and just as importantly, if they are used poorly or incorrectly no harm will be done, and this today is a rare blessing.

To me Edward Bach was a driven genius, guided by firm principles, well-based in the tradition and history of medicine over the centuries. He was also both professionally and personally a saint — the true medical model.

Nora Weeks was for so many years his assistant. Her loving nurture and furtherance of his work after his death has been of great benefit to mankind. Bach's work may not have survived without her. Unlike many other holistic pioneers, Bach was blessed by having Nora Weeks to carry on his work and his message after his death, cementing the foundations so that at the time of her own death, the work is now so well-recognized and well-received that it will never perish nor be forgotten.

Her book is a touching and beautiful tribute to one of the greatest holistic medical pioneers by his loving, dedicated disciple. It is a joy to read and re-read, an inspiration and a guiding light.

John Diamond, M.D.
May, 1979

Bibliography

The Bach Flower Remedies
    Incorporating *Heal Thyself* by Edward Bach, M.D., B.S., D.P.H.; *The Twelve Healers* by Edward Bach, M.D., B.S., D.P.H.; and The Bach Remedies Repertory by F.J. Wheeler, M.D., M.R.C.S., L.R.C.P.
    Published by Keats Publishing, Inc., New Canaan, Connecticut

The Medical Discoveries of Edward Bach, Physician by Nora Weeks, Published by Keats Publishing, Inc.

Handbook of the Bach Flower Remedies by Philip M. Chancellor, Published by Keats Publishing, Inc.

The Bach Flower Remedies — Illustrations and Method of Preparation by Nora Weeks and Victor Bullen. Illustrations by Marjorie Pemberton-Piggott. Published by C.W. Daniel Company, Ltd. London.